The biosynthesis of
secondary
metabolites

THE BIOSYNTHESIS OF SECONDARY METABOLITES

R. B. Herbert
Department of Organic Chemistry
University of Leeds

LONDON NEW YORK
CHAPMAN AND HALL

First published 1981
by Chapman and Hall Ltd
11 New Fetter Lane, London EC4P 4EE
Published in the USA
by Chapman and Hall
in association with Methuen, Inc.
733 Third Avenue, New York, NY 10017
© 1981 R. B. Herbert

Printed and bound in the
United States of America

ISBN 0 412 16370 5 (cased)
ISBN 0 412 16380 2 (paperback)

British Library Cataloguing in Publication Data

Herbert, R. B.
    The biosynthesis of secondary metabolites.
    1. Metabolism, Secondary   2. Biosynthesis
    3. Natural products
    I. Title
    574.19′29   QH521   80-41868

ISBN 0-412-16370-5
ISBN 0-412-16380-2 Pbk

Contents

CONTENTS   vii

TO MY FATHER
on the occasion of his 70th birthday

'I am, in point of fact, a particularly haughty and exclusive person, of pre-Adamite ancestral descent. . . . I can trace my ancestry back to a protoplasmal primordial atomic globule. Consequently my family pride is something inconceivable.'

Pooh-Bah, in *The Mikado*
by W. S. Gilbert and A. Sullivan

Preface

This is a book about experiments and results of experiments. The results described are the fruit of thirty years' labour in the field of secondary metabolism.

Secondary metabolism, more than any other part of the chemistry of life, has been the special preserve of organic chemists. Investigation of secondary metabolism began with curiosity about the structures of compounds isolated from natural sources, i.e. secondary metabolites. Coeval with structure determination there has been a curiosity about the origins and mechanism of formation of secondary metabolites (or natural products as they have been called). It is the experimental outcome of this curiosity that is described here.

This account is primarily intended to be an introduction to the biosynthesis of secondary metabolites. I have also endeavoured, however, to make the book as comprehensive as possible. This has meant that some of the material has had to be presented in abbreviated form. The abbreviated material is largely confined to particular sections of the book. The paragraphs marked with a dagger (†) can be omitted by the reader wishing to acquire a general introduction to the subject.

A blend of the most significant and the most recent references is cited to provide the reader with ready access to the primary literature. This is clearly most necessary for the material presented in abbreviated form. Relevant reviews are also cited.

In compiling this account I am indebted to the following people: Mrs M. Romanowicz for typing the manuscript with accuracy and speed, to my wife, Margaret, for checking the references, to final year Ph.D. students, Stuart H. Hedges and William J. W. Watson for critically reading and checking the typed manuscript, and John E. Cragg for proofreading.

Richard Herbert
June 1980

1. Introduction

1.1 Primary and secondary metabolism

1.1.1 Introduction

Since prehistoric times man has used plant extracts to heal and to kill. Folklore abounds in references to the use of plant extracts in the healing of a variety of illnesses; examples of applications as agents of death range from that of calabar beans and hemlock as judicial poisons to that of the South American curare arrow poisons [1]. In modern times organic compounds isolated from cultures of micro-organisms, as well as from plants, have been used for the cure of disease (e.g. penicillin and tetracycline antibiotics). These organic compounds from natural sources form a large group known as natural products, or secondary metabolites.

Study of the metabolism, fundamental and vital to living things, has led to a detailed understanding of the processes involved. A complex web of enzyme-catalysed reactions is now apparent, which begins with carbon dioxide and photosynthesis and leads to, and beyond, diverse compounds called primary metabolites, e.g. amino acids, acetyl-coenzyme A, mevalonic acid, sugars, and nucleotides [2, 3]. Critical to the overall energetics involved in metabolism is the coenzyme, adenosine triphosphate (ATP), which serves as a common energy relay and co-operates, like other coenzymes, with particular enzymes in the reactions they catalyse.

This intricate web of vital biochemical reactions is referred to as primary metabolism. It is often displayed usefully in chart form [4], and to the eye appears very much like an advanced model railway layout, not least because of the way primary metabolism proceeds in cycles (e.g. the citric acid cycle). The organic compounds of primary metabolism are the stations on the main lines of this railway, the compounds of secondary metabolism the termini of branch lines. Secondary metabolites are distinguished more precisely from primary metabolites by the following criteria: they have a restricted distribution being found mostly in plants and micro-organisms, and are often characteristic of individual genera, species, or strains; they are

1

formed along specialized pathways from primary metabolites. Primary metabolites, by contrast, have a broad distribution in all living things and are intimately involved in essential life processes (for further discussion of parts of primary metabolism see Sections 1.1.2 and 5.1). It follows that secondary metabolites are non-essential to life although they are important to the organism that produces them. What this importance is, however, remains, very largely, obscure.

It is interesting to note that secondary metabolites are biosynthesised essentially from a handful of primary metabolites: α-amino acids, acetyl-coenzyme A, mevalonic acid, and intermediates of the shikimic acid pathway. It is these starting points for the elaboration of secondary metabolites which allow their classification, and also their discussion as discrete groups (Chapters 3 to 7). In the remainder of this chapter various aspects of biosynthesis of general importance to the discussion in Chapter 3 and succeeding chapters is reviewed. The first examples of primary and secondary metabolite biosynthesis will be found in Sections 1.1.2 and 1.1.3. Chapter 2 is devoted to a brief discourse on the various techniques used in studying the biosynthesis of secondary metabolites.

1.1.2 Fatty acid biosynthesis [2, 3]

Fatty acids, e.g. stearic acid (*1.1*) and oleic acid (*1.2*), are straight chain carboxylic acids found predominantly as lipid constituents.

$$CH_3(CH_2)_{16}CO_2H \qquad CH_3(CH_2)_7CH=CH(CH_2)_7CO_2H$$

(1.1) Stearic acid   *(1.2)* Oleic acid

They are primary metabolites formed under enzyme catalysis by linear combination of acetate units. In this they are similar to the polyketides which are secondary metabolites (Chapter 3). Like many primary metabolites, their biosynthesis is understood in intricate detail. Much less detail is generally available on secondary metabolite biosynthesis.

Fatty acids are synthesized in a multienzyme complex from a crucially important primary metabolite, acetyl-coenzyme A (*1.8*). The principal source of acetyl-CoA (*1.8*) is pyruvic acid (*1.5*) and the conversion of (*1.5*) into (*1.8*) involves the coenzymes, thiamine pyrophosphate (*1.3*)* and lipoic acid (*1.6*) (Scheme 1.1). The key to the action of thiamine is the ready formation of the zwitterion (*1.4*) at the beginning and end of the reaction cycle. The lipoic acid (*1.6*) is enzyme linked via the side chain of a lysine residue (*1.7*). The disulphide functionality is thus at the end of a long (14 Å) arm. It has been suggested that this arm allows the lipoate to swing from one

---

* Ⓟ = phosphate in (*1.3*) and subsequent structures, cf. (*1.10*).

(1.3) Thiamine pyrophosphate

(1.4)

(1.5) Pyruvic acid

Coenzyme A
(R—SH)

$CH_3-C-S-R$

Acetyl-coenzyme A
(1.8)

Oxidation

(1.6) R = OH, Lipoic acid

(1.7) R =

Scheme 1.1

site to another within the multienzyme complex and transfer (and oxidize) the acetyl group [5]. In the sequence shown, pyruvic acid (1.5) loses carbon dioxide giving coenzyme-bound acetaldehyde, which is oxidized to the CoA ester of acetic acid.

A similar long arm is apparent in biotin (1.9), again enzyme bound through a lysine residue. The coenzyme (1.9) assists in the carboxylation of acetyl-CoA (1.8) with carbon dioxide yielding malonyl-CoA (1.14). Exchange of both acetyl-CoA and malonyl-CoA occurs with acyl carrier proteins (ACP) having free thiol groupings. Condensation then occurs between acetyl-S-ACP and malonyl-S-ACP with simultaneous decarboxylation; the carboxylate anion is transferred into the new bond (Scheme 1.2) [6]. Subsequent steps involve reduction, dehydration and double-bond saturation. They

(1.9) Biotin

[H]

[H]

(1.10) R = ℗, NADPH
(1.11) R = H, NADH

(1.12) R = ℗, NADP⁺
(1.13) R = H, NAD⁺

implicate in part the widely utilized reducing coenzyme, NADPH (*1.10*) (Scheme 1.2). The first sequence gives butyryl-S-ACP (*1.15*)

$$CH_3-\overset{\overset{O}{\|}}{C}-S \quad CoA \xrightarrow[\text{Biotin}]{CO_2} \quad \overset{\ominus}{\underset{O}{O}}\overset{\overset{O}{\|}}{C}-CH_2-\overset{\overset{O}{\|}}{C}-S-CoA$$

Acetyl-CoA (*1.8*)   (*1.9*)   (*1.14*) Malonyl-CoA

$$CH_3-\overset{\overset{O}{\|}}{C}-S-ACP$$

$$CH_3-\overset{\overset{O}{\|}}{C}-CH_2-\overset{\overset{O}{\|}}{C}-S-ACP$$

NADPH (*1.10*), H$^\oplus$

$$CH_3-\underset{OH}{\overset{|}{C}H}-CH_2-\overset{\overset{O}{\|}}{C}-S-ACP \; + \; NADP^+ \quad (1.12)$$

$$CH_3-CH=CH-\overset{\overset{O}{\|}}{C}-S-ACP$$

NADPH (*1.10*), H$^\oplus$

$$CH_3-CH_2-CH_2-\overset{\overset{O}{\|}}{C}-S-ACP \qquad + \; NADP^+ \quad (1.12)$$

(*1.15*)

Scheme 1.2

and for the generation of longer chains, as (*1.1*), the sequence, of malonyl-CoA addition, reduction, dehydration and reduction, is repeated the requisite number of times.

In examining the overall conversion of pyruvate into a fatty acid (Schemes 1.1 and 1.2) it is interesting to note the exploitation of particular chemical properties of sulphur: (i), as an easily reduced disulphide (*1.6*); (ii), as an easily oxidized dithiol; and (iii) in reactive thioesters which aid the Claisen-type condensation reactions. Also of crucial importance for the condensation is the use of a malonic acid derivative (*1.14*) as a source of a stable anion. (Further discussion of fatty acid biosynthesis in relation to polyketide formation is taken up in Chapter 3.)

1.1.3 The biosynthesis of polyacetylenes and prostaglandins
The formation of unsaturated fatty acids, e.g. oleic acid (*1.2*), which are also primary metabolites, may occur by at least two routes, one aerobic the other anaerobic. Essentially though, both involve desaturation of a fully saturated fatty acid [2]. Polyacetylenes, e.g. crepenynic acid (*1.16*), which are secondary metabolites, also

apparently derive by step-wise desaturation of a saturated fatty acid [7]. The path to crepenynic acid (*1.16*) is illustrated in Scheme 1.3.

$$(1.1) \rightarrow (1.2) \rightarrow CH_3(CH_2)_4 \, CH=CHCH_2CH=CH(CH_2)_7 \, CO_2H$$

$$CH_3(CH_2)_4 \, C\equiv CCH_2CH=CH(CH_2)_7 \, CO_2H$$

(*1.16*) Crepenynic acid

Scheme 1.3

Prostaglandins, e.g. prostaglandin E_2 (*1.19*), are physiologically active secondary metabolites found in mammals. The biosynthesis of these compounds also involves an unsaturated fatty acid, e.g. arachidonic acid (*1.17*). Formation of the characteristic prostaglandin skeleton involves the formation of an intermediate endoperoxide (*1.18*). Some of the succeeding steps are indicated in Scheme 1.4 [8–10].

(*1.17*)

(*1.19*) Prostaglandin E_2 (*1.18*)

Scheme 1.4

It is interesting to note the formation of polyacetylenes (and prostaglandins) from fatty acids, since it is unusual for secondary metabolites to be formed from a fatty acid. The route that dominates the formation of these metabolites is the polyketide one (Chapter 3).

1.2 Stereochemistry and biosynthesis

1.2.1 Chirality and prochirality [11]

It is a common observation that enzymes deal stereospecifically with their substrates; the acceptable substrates must have a particular stereochemistry and the products in turn are formed with a particular stereochemistry (for an illustration of this see particularly Section 5.1). This stereospecificity is associated in many instances with reactions involving chiral centres.

In addition to the stereospecificity of reaction associated with chiral centres there is further stereospecificity to be found in reactions at prochiral centres. The conversion of ethanol (*1.20*) into acetaldehyde (*1.21*) by the enzyme, alcohol dehydrogenase, with NAD^+ as co-enzyme provides a simple illustration. The methylene group in (*1.20*) is prochiral*. Oxidation of the ethanol proceeds stereospecifically with removal of the *pro-R* proton from this group. The reverse reaction involves stereospecific addition of a proton to the *re*-face (in this case, the top face as seen by the reader) of the acetaldehyde carbonyl group (i.e. proton removal and addition to the same side of the two molecules). The reaction is, moreover, stereospecific with regard to coenzyme. The interconversion of NADH and NAD$^+$ involves, respectively, removal of a proton from a prochiral centre and proton addition to form one. Removal and addition again involves the same face of the molecules concerned.

Scheme 1.5

The stereospecific proton removal from (*1.20*) to give (*1.21*) can be understood simply as follows: Imagine that at the active site of the enzyme there is one binding site specific for the ethanol OH and one specific for CH$_3$. This uniquely locates the molecules on the enzyme surface as shown in (*1.20*). Now imagine that the enzyme/co-enzyme proton removal can only occur physically from above the plane of the paper. This results in unique removal of the *pro-R* proton. There is no way on this model that the *pro-S* proton can be removed. A similar argument can be applied to proton addition to (*1.21*) and to

---

*The methylene group of ethanol has two identical groups (H) on a tetrahedral carbon atom and two groups different from these and from each other (CH$_3$, OH), and so is *pro*-chiral: a single change in one of the identical groups (H) makes the centre *chiral*. The identical groups may be distinguished as *pro-R* and *pro-S*. In order to do this the priority of one of the identical groups (H) is raised over the other. If this is done for the hydrogen projecting above the plane of the paper in (*1.20*) then the configuration at the methylene carbon atom becomes *R*. So the hydrogen that is raised in priority is termed *pro-R*. [The reader can try labelling the carboxy-methyl groups in (*1.22*) similarly; answer: (*1.60*).] The acetaldehyde double bond is also prochiral: the two faces of the double bond are not identical (addition may give a chiral product). These faces may be labelled *re* and *si* by following the normal priority rules for chirality (*re* = *R*, *si* = *S*). The face of (*1.21*) viewed from above is *re* (for further discussion see [12]).

(1.22) Citric acid

proton removal from, and addition to, co-enzyme. [This argument was first applied some thirty years ago to citric acid *(1.22)* in relation to its place in the citric acid cycle. Citric acid has a prochiral centre (*) [13].]

1.2.2 Chiral methyl groups [14]

Enzyme reactions involving methyl groups show none of the stereochemistry associated with prochiral centres as, e.g., the methylene group in ethanol (see above). The hydrogen atoms are indistinguishable (provided they are all one hydrogen isotope, see below) but enzyme-catalysed reactions do occur which involve methyl groups in various ways. Since enzymes are involved the reactions are expected to proceed with a particular stereochemistry. Three main classes of reaction can be identified [14]. By way of illustration we shall briefly examine one of these (Scheme 1.6) (for

Isopentenyl pyrophosphate   Dimethylallyl pyrophosphate

Scheme 1.6

further discussion see Section 4.4). Proton addition to C^* of the double bond in *(1.23)*, with formation of a methyl group, can, in principle, occur from above or below the plane of the double bond. If the three protons involved in the generation of the methyl group are labelled with the three isotopes of hydrogen [^{1}H, ^{2}H, and ^{3}H, indicated in Scheme 1.7 as, respectively, H, D, and T] then the methyl

Scheme 1.7

group generated will be chiral. The stereochemical course of the reaction can be deduced, provided that: (i), the chirality (*R* or *S*) of the asymmetric methyl group thus generated can be determined; and

(ii), the substitution of hydrogen isotope around the double bond in
(1.24) is known, e.g. as shown.

The central analytical problem is to determine the chirality of
methyl groups generated or modified in biochemical reactions. The
solution is dazzlingly ingenious. First, samples of chiral acetic acid
[as (1.26)] of known absolute configuration were synthesized. All
molecules of acetic acid contained deuterium (and hydrogen) but, as
is customary, only very few molecules were also labelled with
tritium. Only very few molecules were therefore chiral. Since the
analysis is for tritium, however, this does not matter. [Subsequently
an economical and supremely elegant synthesis of chiral acetic acid
has been developed (Scheme 1.8), which involves two stereospecific

Scheme 1.8

concerted reactions and transfer of the chirality in (1.25) into (1.26)
[15].]

The method of analysis developed is for acetic acid and involves
the use of two enzymes. Chiral acetic acid [as (1.26)] is irreversibly
condensed as its CoA-derivative with glyoxylic acid (1.27), using the
enzyme malate synthase, to give malic acid (1.28). The condensation
occurs with loss of hydrogen isotope by a primary kinetic isotope
effect ($k_H > k_D > k_T$). This means that loss of H is favoured over loss
of D which is in turn favoured over loss of T. The result is a high
retention of tritium.

By loss of deuterium (^2H) or protium (^1H) two samples of *radioactive* malate are formed: (1.28) as major product by loss of H, and
(1.29) as minor product from (R)-acetic acid by loss of ^2H (D);
(1.33) and (1.34) are, respectively, the major and minor radioactive
products from (S)-acetic acid (1.32). (The malate synthase reaction
is now known to proceed with inversion of configuration. Since the
method of analysis depends on simply getting one result for R-acetic
acid and the opposite for the S-isomer this does not matter for the
purposes of *assay*.)

(1.27)   *(1.28)* Malic acid   *(1.30)* Fumaric acid

Major isomer

Minor isomer

(1.29)   *(1.31)*

(1.32) (S)–Acetic acid   *(1.33)* Major isomer   *(1.34)* Minor isomer

Scheme 1.9

The malic acid is isolated and incubated with fumarase until no further loss of carbon-bound tritium results. [The enzyme catalyses *trans* removal of water, as *(1.28)* ⇌ *(1.30)*.] For the samples of malate derived from (*R*)-acetic acid, the minor product *(1.29)* loses TOH. For the material derived from (*S*)-acetic acid it is the major product *(1.33)* which loses TOH. So for (*R*)-acetic acid a higher retention of tritium (ca. 75%) is observed in the fumarase equilibration and for (*S*)-acetic acid a lower value (ca. 25%). With the method of analysis established for samples of acetic acid of known chirality it can be used to determine the configuration of samples of acetic acid of unknown chirality derived from biological reactions (for examples see Section 4.2 and 4.4, and [14]).

1.2.3 *Hydroxylation at saturated carbon atoms* [2]

An oft encountered reaction in secondary metabolite biosynthesis is hydroxylation at saturated carbon atoms. These reactions are mediated by a mixed-function oxidase (or mono-oxygenase) i.e. an oxidase which uses molecular oxygen for hydroxylation, according to the equation: substrate-H + O_2 + XH_2 → substrate-OH + H_2O + X.

These hydroxylations are stereospecific proceeding with retention of configuration [11, 16] (examples are cited in following Chapters). This is the expected result for an electrophilic substitution at saturated carbon, i.e. attack at the point of highest electron density which is the sigma bond itself [17].

1.3 Some reactions of general importance in secondary metabolism

It will be convenient to discuss under this heading three quite different reaction types which will be mentioned again in succeeding
chapters. Two concern aromatic compounds only, the third is of
widespread significance.

1.3.1 *Oxidative coupling of phenols* [18–20]

Phenols are biosynthesized essentially in two ways. One is along the
polyketide pathway starting with acetyl-CoA (Chapter 3), the other
along the shikimic acid pathway (Chapter 5). A phenol, or indeed
any benzenoid compound, so formed may be at a terminus in biosynthesis or be involved in the formation of other metabolites. Of general importance in this regard is the coupling together of two
phenolic residues, e.g. *(1.35)* → *(1.38)*. A firm mechanistic base was
given to this process by the quite brilliant recognition that this bond
forming could occur by inter- or intra-molecular coupling of two
mesomeric radicals [as *(1.36)*] formed by the one-electron oxidation
of each of a pair of phenols. Carbon–carbon bond formation can
only occur, according to this hypothesis, *ortho* or *para* to the phenolic
hydroxy groups. Numerous studies on the biosynthesis of various
phenolic compounds (see Sections 6.2.2, 6.3, 6.4 and 3.3) have
demonstrated the overall correctness of this hypothesis: coupling is
always *ortho* or *para* to phenolic hydroxy groups (occasionally
C—O—C bonds may be formed); a hydroxy group must always be
present on each of the aromatic rings (*O*-alkylation, for instance,
blocks the coupling reaction). In one exceptional case (Section 6.3.5)
it has been found that coupling only occurs if one of the aromatic
rings bears *two* hydroxy functions.

Chemical conversion of *p*-cresol into the ketone *(1.39)* provides a
simple illustration of the hypothesis (Scheme 1.10), in which coupling occurs between the position *ortho* to one phenolic hydroxy group

Scheme 1.10

and the position *para* to the other. Aromaticity is regained by proton loss from the coupling sites(s) [as $(1.37) \rightarrow (1.38)$ and $(1.42) \rightarrow (1.43)$]. In the formation of (1.38) only one ring can become

(1.42)   (1.43)

aromatic in this way; the methyl group in the other ring secures it in the dienone form (1.38). Such dienones have been isolated from living things. They may react in the way shown for $(1.38) \rightarrow (1.39)$. A strikingly close analogue of (1.39) is the plant alkaloid lunarine (1.41). It arises plausibly from two molecules of *p*-hydroxycinnamic acid (1.40) along a pathway similar to that shown for (1.39). [In support, phenylalanine, a precursor for (1.40), is incorporated into lunarine (1.41) [21].]

Instead of undergoing a ring-closure reaction of the type just described, dienones may rearrange *in vivo* [as $(1.44) \rightarrow (1.45)$] and thus regain aromaticity (the 'dienone-phenol' rearrangement). Reduction gives dienols [as (1.46)] which either rearrange [as $(1.46) \rightarrow (1.48)$ ('dienol-benzene' rearrangement)] or undergo ring-closure reactions of the type $(1.46) \rightarrow (1.47)$. An outstanding example of the latter reaction involving a dienol is found in the biosynthesis of morphine (Section 6.3.4), and of the former in the biosynthesis of isothebaine (Section 6.3.2). (The various possibilities are summarized in Schemes 1.10 and 1.11; *ortho-para* coupling is illustrated; similar schemes can be written for *ortho-ortho* and *para-para* coupling.)

Scheme 1.11

1.3.2 *Hydroxylation of aromatic substrates* [22, 23]

It has been found generally in a variety of living systems that hydroxylation of aromatic substrates involves utilization of molecular oxygen and proceeds *via* an arene oxide [as *(1.49)*]. Collapse of this arene oxide to give *(1.51)* occurs with a 1,2 shift of the substituent X (e.g. X = ^1H, ^2H, ^3H, Cl). In the hydroxylation of 4'-chlorophenylalanine *(1.52)* proton loss occurs from *(1.50)* to give 3'-chloro-4'-hydroxyphenylalanine *(1.54)* as the major product. For X = ^3H (T) or ^2H (D) loss of hydrogen isotope occurs from *(1.50)* in accord with a primary isotope effect ($k_H > k_D > k_T$). Thus hydroxylation of [4'-^3H]phenylalanine *(1.53)* gives the α-amino acid tyrosine *(1.55)* with a high retention (ca. 90%) of tritium at C-3'. A lower retention is observed for [4'-^2H]phenylalanine (ca. 70%) as a reflection of the different isotope effects. This 1,2-shift in aromatic hydroxylation is called the NIH shift (named after the National Institutes of Health, U.S.A., where the rearrangement was discovered).

Subsequent hydroxylation of tyrosine [as *(1.55)*] to give dopa [as *(1.56)*] occurs without NIH shift, i.e. loss of substituent X, although another arene oxide is probably implicated. For the conversion of [4'-^3H]phenylalanine *(1.53)* → *(1.55)* → *(1.56)*, ca. 90% tritium is retained after the first hydroxylation. Half of this is lost in the next reaction because there are two equivalent (C-3' and C-5') sites, each bearing half of the residual tritium, which are available in *(1.55)* for oxygenation and consequent loss of tritium.

1.3.3 Methylation [2]

C-, *O*-, and *N*-methylations are encountered frequently in the biosynthesis of secondary metabolites. All appear to involve nucleophilic substitution on the *S*-methyl group of *S*-adenosyl-L-methionine *(1.59)* (Scheme 1.12). In biosynthetic feeding experiments it is normal to use [*methyl*-^{14}C]methionine [as *(1.58)*] as a precursor for methyl groups; reaction *in vivo* with ATP and Mg^{2+} affords *(1.59)*. Particu-

(1.49)   *(1.50)*   *(1.51)*

(1.52) X = Cl   *(1.54)* X = Cl   *(1.56)*
(1.53) X = T   *(1.55)* X = T

(1.57)   *(1.58)* Methionine   *(1.59)* S-Adenosylmethionine

Scheme 1.12

(1.60)

larly in early studies formic acid was used to test for C_1 units in biosynthesis. It serves as a source for methyl groups via N-formyltetrahydrofolic acid which suffers reduction to give N-methyltetrahydrofolic acid; the methyl group is then transferred to L-homocysteine (1.57) to give L-methionine (1.58).

References

Further reading: [2] and [3].

[1] Swan, G. A. (1967), *An Introduction to the Alkaloids*, Blackwell Scientific Publications, Oxford.
[2] Mahler, H. R and Cordes, E. H. (1971), *Biological Chemistry*, 2nd Edn, Harper and Row, New York.
[3] Staunton, J. (1978), *Primary Metabolism: a mechanistic approach*, Clarendon Press, Oxford.
[4] Dagley, S. and Nicholson, D. E. (1970), *An Introduction to Metabolic Pathways*, Blackwell Scientific Publications, Oxford.
[5] Reed, L. J. (1974), *Acc. Chem. Res.*, **7**, 40–6.
[6] Arnstadt, K.-I., Schindlbeck, G. and Lynen, F. (1975), *Eur. J. Biochem.*, **55**, 561–71.
[7] Bu'Lock, J. D. and Smith, G. N. (1967), *J. Chem. Soc. (C)*, 332–6.
[8] Bergström, S. (1967), *Science*, **157**, 382–91.
[9] Hamberg, M., Svensson, J., Wakabayashi, T. and Samuelsson, B. (1974), *Proc. Natl. Acad. Sci. U.S.A.*, **71**, 345–9.
[10] Hamberg, M., Svensson, J. and Samuelsson, B. (1975), *Proc. Natl. Acad. Sci. U.S.A.*, **72**, 2994–8.
[11] Bentley, R. (1969), *Molecular Asymmetry in Biology*, Academic Press, Vol. 1; (1970), vol. 2.
[12] Hanson, K. R. (1966), *J. Am. Chem. Soc.*, **88**, 2731–42.
[13] Ogston, A. G. (1948), *Nature*, **162**, 963.
[14] Cornforth, J. W. (1970), *Chem. in Brit.*, **6**, 431–6.
[15] Townsend, C. A., Scholl, T. and Arigoni, D. (1975), *J. Chem. Soc. Chem. Comm.*, 921–2.
[16] Battersby, A. R., Staunton, J., Wiltshire, H. R., Bircher, B. J. and Fuganti, C. (1975), *J. Chem. Soc. Perkin 1*, 1162–71; and their ref. 11.
[17] Olah, G. (1972), *Chem. in Brit.*, **8**, 281–7.
[18] Barton, D. H. R. and Cohen, T. (1957), in *Festschrift Dr A. Stoll*, Birkhaüser, Basle, pp. 117–43.
[19] Erdtman, H. and Wachtmeister, C. A. (1957), in *Festschrift Dr A. Stoll*, Birkhaüser, Basle, pp. 144–65.
[20] Taylor, W. 1. and Battersby, A. R. (eds.) (1967), *Oxidative Coupling of Phenols*, Arnold, London.

[21] Poupat, C. and Kunesch, G. (1971), *Compt. rend.*, **273C**, 433–6.
[22] Auret, B. J., Boyd, D. R., Robinson, P. M., Watson, C. G., Daly, J. W. and Jerina, D. M. (1971), *J. Chem. Soc. Chem. Comm.*, 1585–7.
[23] Guroff, G., Daly, J. W., Jerina, D. M., Renson, J., Witkop, B. and Udenfriend, S. (1967), *Science*, **157**, 1524–30.

2. Techniques for biosynthesis

2.1 Introduction

In the study of secondary metabolism the ongoing problem is two-fold: (i), to identify the source(s) in primary metabolism from which a secondary metabolite has its genesis; and (ii), to identify by what mechanisms and manner of intermediates it is thus fashioned. It is structure that first hints at a solution made complete by a battery of special techniques.

The biosynthetic pathway by which a primary metabolite is formed may be an intricate one involving complex chemistry. Thus the structure of a primary metabolite does not necessarily yield any immediate clues to its mode of biosynthesis (see, e.g., the biosynthesis of the α-amino acid, tyrosine, in Section 5.1). By contrast the structure of a secondary metabolite often allows accurate speculation about its origins and even its mechanism of formation. Such speculation has long been the hand-maid of structure determination, e.g. consideration of the possible biogenesis of the alkaloid, morphine, indicated the correct structure (*2.2*) for it in the midst of confusing chemical evidence. Both the isoprene rule (Chapter 4) and the polyketide hypothesis (Chapter 3), underpinned by coherent biogenetic speculation, have been, and continue to be, invaluable in the structure determination of natural products. They are based on the fact that large numbers of secondary metabolites are formed from one or two simple repeating units.

It is because, in the event, secondary metabolites derive from but a handful of primary metabolites along pathways involving generally the simplest reactions in organic chemistry and little rearrangement, that speculation about their biosynthesis can be so accurate. Also invaluable in this regard, is the identification of metabolites of similar structure in the same, or related, species. Thus benzyl-isoquinoline alkaloids [as (*2.1*)] and morphine (*2.2*) are both found in *Papaver* species. It follows reasonably that morphine derives from a compound type of (*2.1*) (Section 6.3.4).

The wealth of intelligent speculation about the biosynthesis of secondary metabolites has provided a firm base from which to mount

Tyrosine   (2.1) Reticuline   (2.2) Morphine

wide-ranging experimental forays into secondary metabolism in search of origins and mechanism of formation. The experiments are carried out using a variety of techniques. The dominant technique involves the administration of likely precursors to an organism, and examination of the secondary metabolite produced to see if the compounds 'fed' were used in the formation of the metabolite. In this way, tyrosine and (2.1) have been shown to be involved in morphine biosynthesis. To track the likely precursor through to the metabolite, the precursor must be labelled, or marked, in some way. A variety of 'labels' are used. First, there are radioactive isotopic labels, e.g. ^{14}C and ^{3}H (tritium) which are very sensitively assayed by scintillation counting (Section 2.2.1) (tyrosine was examined as a morphine precursor with a ^{14}C label at C-2). Second, there are stable isotopic labels, e.g. ^{13}C, ^{15}N, ^{18}O, ^{2}H (deuterium) which are very much less sensitively assayed by mass spectrometry and, for some, n.m.r. spectroscopy (Section 2.2.2).

In addition to the results of feeding experiments with labelled precursors, clear information on the sequence of biosynthesis of several related metabolites produced by an organism may be obtained. This is done by feeding a very early precursor (usually $^{14}CO_2$) and noting the order in which the metabolites are labelled. This order gives the sequence of biosynthesis.

Experiments with purified enzymes involved in biosynthesis, or even experiments with crude enzyme preparations, can provide important definition of a pathway. Studies with enzymes are briefly referred to, by way of introduction, in Section 2.3, as is the use of mutants.

It is usually a simple matter to feed a micro-organism, growing in liquid culture, with a labelled precursor. Commonly aqueous solutions are added at predetermined time(s) to the culture and the metabolite is isolated and purified some time later. It is more difficult to feed precursors to plants. A variety of methods are used: (i), a wick is threaded through the lower part of the plant stem and dipped into an aqueous solution of the precursor: (ii), assimilation through the roots by standing the plant in an aqueous solution of the precursor; (iii), injection into a hollow stem or seed capsule; and (iv), standing excised parts of the plant in an aqueous solution of the precursor.

In feeding experiments with labelled precursors common problems arise.

(i) A very reasonable precursor may be utilized in metabolite biosynthesis at a very low level or not at all. This may be: (a), because of the difficulty in getting the precursor to the site of biosynthesis (a perennial problem), or (b), because it is genuinely not involved in the biosynthesis of the chosen metabolite, or (c), because it is used much more efficiently for the formation of another secondary, or primary, metabolite. A further problem, in studies with plants, is that the particular metabolite might not be undergoing biosynthesis at the time of the experiment. Thus a negative result with a labelled precursor is always ambiguous, never certain.

(ii) Even if a labelled compound, (C in 2.3) is shown to be an efficient precursor* for a metabolite, D, it does not mean it is an obligatory intermediate in the biosynthesis of D. It may just have been a convenient foreign substrate dealt with economically by the living system. However, if the precursor, C, can be shown to occur in the organism under examination and be formed like the metabolite, D, from the same earlier precursor(s), e.g. A, then it is most likely to be a true intermediate. Its status as an intermediate can be further strengthened by the appropriate experiments with enzymes isolated from the living system.

(iii) The precursor may be at a shunt (E) from the main pathway (A → B → C → D) in (2.3). It is difficult to resolve whether or not

$$A \longrightarrow B \longrightarrow C \longrightarrow D$$
$$\qquad \updownarrow \qquad \text{Metabolite}$$
$$\qquad E$$
$$(2.3)$$

this is so and final conclusions depend on the balance of the evidence.

2.2 Isotopic labelling
Simple compounds bearing isotopic labels can be bought. More complex compounds must be synthesized [8].

---

*The efficiency with which a precursor is utilized is given either by the percentage of label incorporated from the precursor into the metabolite or by the extent to which the precursor label is diluted in the derived metabolite. It is normal to compare the values for several precursors: efficiency is only really significant in a relative sense. A precursor earlier in a pathway will normally be incorporated less efficiently and with higher dilution (passing through more metabolic pools) than one which appears later. Acceptable incorporations in plants are often below 1%, but experiments with microorganisms usually return acceptable incorporations above 1%.

2.2.1   Radioactive isotopes

Tritium (^{3}H) and ^{14}C, with half-lives of 12.26 years and 5600 years respectively, are the most commonly used radioactive isotopes. They are used extensively to monitor the uptake of precursors into metabolites and to determine the fates of individual hydrogens or carbons in a precursor during biosynthesis. Tritium finds particular application in this latter regard because any number of proton additions/removals and rearrangements may occur in the course of the biotransformation of precursor into metabolite. (Tritium loss is normally measured by reference to a ^{14}C label in the precursor which is known not to be lost during biosynthesis.)

The isotopes, ^{14}C and ^{3}H, are both β-emitters. They are assayed by liquid scintillation counting. In simple terms, the method involves dissolving the radioactive compound in a scintillant 'cocktail' containing phosphors which convert the β-radiation into light. The light emitted is measured within the scintillation counter by photomultiplier tubes and is expressed as counts against time, a normal way of expressing radioactivity. In practice radioactivity is measured within the counter at less than 100% efficiency. The actual efficiency must be determined and allowance made for this in calculating the true activity of the sample (in decompositions $\sec^{-1}$ mmol^{-1}; 1 Curie = 3.7×10^{10} d $\sec^{-1}$). Reliable radioactivity measurements depend: (i), on recrystallization of the sample, or a derivative, to constant radioactivity; and (ii), on obtaining counts for the radioactive compound at twice the value for an inactive (background) sample (this is the lower limit for radioactivity measurement).

The fate of radioactive labels, particularly carbon, is determined by unambiguous degradation of the radioactive metabolite to isolate the labelling site from all others. Specific labelling of a particular site, or sites, indicates specific utilization of the precursor, e.g [1-^{14}C]acetic acid (2.4) specifically labels the sites indicated in orsellinic acid (2.5), thus showing that acetic acid is specifically a source for

(2.5), and that it is used in the way shown. Spread of acetate radioactivity, say, over all the carbon atoms in (2.5) would clearly indicate fragmentation of the precursor before utilization in the biosynthesis of (2.5). Without determination of the site of labelling the real significance of the measured incorporation of a precursor, which could be due either to specific, or to random, incorporation, would remain unknown.

It is possible for a fairly complex precursor to suffer *partial* fragmentation prior to use. Use of a single label and even showing that the label is specifically at the expected site may well not reveal this. So intact incorporation is more accurately established by using a precursor with labels in two sites as distant as possible from each other. The precursor can only be incorporated into the metabolite intact if the ratio between the two labels in precursor and metabolite is maintained. If once two fragments are formed, each bearing a single label, the chances are remote that they will recombine from the metabolic pools in the living system to give another precursor with the same ratio of labels. Two ^{14}C labels may be used in this sort of experiment but it is simpler to use a ^{14}C and a ^3H label. A notable example is to be found in the biosynthesis of mesembrine alkaloids where the use of doubly labelled precursors indicated their fragmentation where singly labelled precursors indicated intact incorporation (Section 6.4.2).

Although ^{14}C and ^3H, are both β-emitters, ^3H is fortunately a lower energy β-emitter than ^{14}C and there are sufficient differences in their energy spectra to enable one to obtain a separate estimate of the amount of ^{14}C and ^3H a molecule contains.

Unlike stable isotopes radioactive ones are generally only present in compounds at very low enrichment, i.e. the bulk of the material is non-radioactive.

When using a mixture of labels, e.g. ^{14}C and ^3H, it is normal to prepare the compounds with single labels and then mix them. Because of the low enrichment of isotopic label in a compound it is most unlikely that a *single molecule* of, e.g., a multiply labelled species will, in any case, have more than one site labelled, i.e. [(2.6); labels as shown] is made up of (2.7), (2.8) and (2.9). So also, for example, ethanol tritiated on C-1 is made up of (2.10), (2.11) and (2.12).

Normal chemical removal of a hydrogen atom from C-1 will result in loss of ^1H rather than ^3H, by a primary kinetic isotope effect, i.e. high tritium retention: ca. 90%. Stereospecific hydrogen removal from the methylene group will not be influenced by the isotope effect and will result in removal of ^{3}H from (2.11) and ^{1}H from (2.12), or *vice versa*, i.e. 50% retention of tritium. A 50% tritium retention, i.e. sterospecificity, in such a system during biosynthesis indicates an enzyme-catalysed reaction. [For further discussion of reactions at centres like that of the methylene group in (2.10) and the associated stereochemistry see Section 1.2.1.] The actual stereochemistry of this and other reactions can be probed by employing the individual, chirally labelled, molecules [as (2.11) and (2.12)]. One species will suffer complete loss of tritium in a stereospecific (enzyme-catalysed) reaction, the other complete retention. If the chirality of the fed material is known then the stereochemical course of the reaction follows. Numerous applications are to be found in following chapters. The most outstanding are in the complex area of steroid biosynthesis (Chapter 4) where brilliant use has been made of chirally tritiated mevalonic acid samples to determine the intricate detail of biosynthesis.

Use of the three isotopes of hydrogen to fabricate chiral methyl groups for study of the stereochemistry of enzyme-catalysed reactions involving methyl groups is to be noted (Sections 1.2.2, 4.2 and 4.4).

Although radioactive isotopes are used commonly in trace amounts, tritium if present in high concentration can be measured as an n.m.r. signal, e.g. in the biosynthesis of cycloartenol (Section 4.2). Information about the location and stereochemistry of a tritium label was immediately apparent from the n.m.r. spectrum which would not have been the case with scintillation counting.

2.2.2 Stable isotopes

Stable isotopes can yield more information more quickly than radioactive ones. Although rapidly applied, the methods of analysis (n.m.r. spectroscopy and mass spectrometry) are much less sensitive than the method used to assay radioactivity. So a high enrichment is necessary and much more precursor needs to be fed. There is thus a real danger of so much being administered that the normal metabolism of the organism under study is disturbed, resulting in false conclusions. This is not the case with radioactive precursors because they are almost always fed in trace amounts with minimum disturbance of normal metabolism.

All organic molecules contain a significant amount of ^{13}C (natural abundance: 1.1% of ^{12}C) and much lesser amounts of ^{2}H (natural abundance: 0.015%) and, where relevant, ^{15}N (natural abundance: 0.36%). The presence of naturally abundant stable isotopes within a molecule ultimately limits the amount of precursor label which can be detected in a metabolite. This is particularly true where ^{13}C, the most abundant isotope, is involved. Enhanced signals in the ^{13}C n.m.r. spectrum of a metabolite formed from a labelled precursor indicates the location of the label. A lower practical limit for accurate estimation is a signal enriched to the extent of 20% over the natural abundance signal; in practice much higher enrichments are sought for accuracy. Similar problems in estimating low enrichment are encountered in mass spectrometric analysis. Any single ^{13}C, ^2H or ^{15}N label has to be measured on the $M + 1$ peak. The natural abundance peak can be quite intense, e.g. $C_{10}H_{12}$ shows $M + 1$ of 11% of M^+. Thus accurate estimation of small increments in intensity will be difficult. If more than one $^{13}C/^2H/^{15}N$ is present this difficulty is alleviated since for, e.g., $C_{10}H_{12}$, $M + 2$, the peak to be measured if two stable isotopes are present, has an intensity of only 0.6%.

It is generally true that precursors are incorporated into plant metabolites at a low level (of the order of 1% or less) and with high dilution of label. Because of this, and the insensitivity of the methods of analysis for stable isotopes, few experiments have been carried out in plants using them [9, 10].

A significant advantage of stable isotopes over radioactive ones resides in the high enrichment (approaching 100%) of stable isotopes used. It is a simple thing to have two or more labels within the *same* precursor molecule (cf. by contrast, radioactive labels, above). The advantages will be apparent in the ensuing discussion (see also following chapters).

In particular cases it is necessary to determine the origins or fate of oxygen in biosynthesis. For this only the stable ^{18}O isotope (natural abundance: 0.2%) is available and it is analysed for by mass spectrometry, a single ^{18}O label giving rise to $M + 2$ peaks which are measured with comparative sensitivity. The stable isotopes, ^{13}C, ^{15}N, and ^2H (deuterium), can be analysed for similarly, but also by n.m.r. spectroscopy which has found the widest application in ^{13}C assay [3–7].

The first requirement in using ^{13}C labelling for studying the biosynthesis of a particular compound is to assign the resonances in the natural abundance ^{13}C n.m.r. spectrum of the metabolite. Any mistakes in assignment can lead to false conclusions about biosynthesis as, for example, in aflatoxin biosynthesis (Section 3.8). Incorporation of ^{13}C label from a precursor leads to enhanced n.m.r. signals in the metabolite derived from it. Multicolic acid (*2.15*) biosynthesized from [^{13}C]acetate provides one example [11] among many [3–6]. Enhanced n.m.r. signals in (*2.16*) for C-1, C-3, C-5, C-7, C-9, and C-10 from [2-^{13}C]acetate and complementary results with [1-^{13}C]acetate outline the precursor labelling pattern.

More powerfully still, as mentioned above, one may use precursors with two or more labels within the *same* molecule. Thus use of [1,2-$^{13}C_2$]acetate has revolutionized the study of polyketide biosynthesis

(Chapter 3). This dilabelled acetate is normally assimilated into a metabolite under conditions where it will be formed from the labelled precursor after dilution by the organisms' own unlabelled acetate. The metabolite will then be formed very largely, if not completely, so that no two labelled acetate units are adjacent to one another. In the n.m.r. spectrum of the metabolite, coupling will now be seen between the signals for the ^{13}C labels of intact acetate units, and these only. So in the spectrum of (2.16), derived from [^{13}C$_2$]acetate, coupling may be discerned between C-8 and C-9, C-7 and C-6, C-5 and C-2, C-10 and C-4, but C-1, C-3, and C-11 appear as singlets. So C-10, C-4, C-2, and C-5 through C-9 represent intact acetate units (see thickened bonds) and C-1, C-3, and C-11 fragmented ones. The likely biosynthesis of multicolic acid (2.15) follows as shown in Scheme 2.1.

Scheme 2.1

Another example using [1,2-^{13}C$_2$]acetate is provided by mollisin (2.18) where uncertainty prevailed about its pattern of biosynthesis from multiples of acetic acid arising from available ^{14}C data. [1,2-^{13}C$_2$]Acetate (2.13) gave mollisin (2.18), the ^{13}C n.m.r. spectrum of which showed doublets superimposed on natural abundance singlets for all signals except those for C-1 and C-11 which were enhanced singlets. C-1 and C-11 thus derive from fragmented acetate units and the pattern of biosynthesis follows as shown in (2.17) [12]. (For further discussion see Section 3.7.)

A different approach to the use of a precursor with two adjacent ^{13}C atoms in this way, is one in which a precursor is labelled on two atoms expected to come together in the course of biosynthesis. Coupling in the n.m.r. spectrum of the derived metabolite indicates that these atoms have indeed become contiguous. For example, a re-arrangement occurs in the conversion of phenylalanine (2.19) into tropic acid (2.20) (Section 6.2.2). [1,3-^{13}C$_2$]Phenylalanine [as (2.19), labels in the same molecule] gave tropic acid (2.20) in which coupling was observed between C-1 and C-2, thus proving that rearrangement occurs by an intra-molecular 1,2-shift of the phenylalanine carboxy group. (Inter-molecular rearrangement would have given species

(2.19) → (2.20)

(2.21)

labelled on either C-1 or C-2 but not on both as a result of dilution in metabolic pools.) For a further important example (in porphyrin biosynthesis) see [13, 14]

A technically advanced application of ^{13}C n.m.r. spectroscopy is to be found in a study of porphyrin biosynthesis. The course of an enzymatic conversion has been studied by carrying out the reaction in an n.m.r. sample tube, with precursor judiciously labelled with ^{13}C [15].

^{15}N is the isotope of nitrogen available for biosynthetic studies. Its use as a label in α-amino acids does not always give reliable results because of ready transamination in these compounds. ^{15}N may be analysed for by mass spectrometry and also, more recently, by ^{15}N n.m.r. spectroscopy (see, e.g. [16, 17]). It may also find application in conjunction with ^{13}C. In the biosynthesis of a microbial metabolite, streptonigrin (Section 7.5.4) precursor bond cleavage could, *a priori*, have occurred on either side (a or b) of the ring nitrogen atom in tryptophan (2.21). Maintenance of ^{15}N–^{13}C coupling in the ^{13}C n.m.r. spectrum of streptonigrin derived from [1′-^{15}N, 2′-^{13}C]tryptophan indicated clearly that bond cleavage is along dotted line b in (2.21).

Deuterium (^2H) is the stable isotope of hydrogen. It may be analysed for by mass spectrometry and also by the absence of signals in proton n.m.r. spectra. Most recently deuterium has been analysed for directly by ^2H n.m.r. spectroscopy [7]. A particular method of analysis (Section 4.4) involves the measurement of optical activity in deuteriated succinic acid samples as a means of probing the stereochemistry of a biosynthetic sequence [18].

An interesting application of mixed ^{13}C, ^2H labelling is in a study of fusicoccin (2.27) biosynthesis. At the beginning of the study it was known that C-3, C-7, C-11, and C-15 were labelled by [3-^{13}C]mevalonate (2.22) and that three out of a possible four 4-(*R*)-mevalonoid protons (shown circled) were retained on formation of the fusicoccin skeleton (2.27). A plausible route involved cyclization of geranylgeranyl pyrophosphate (2.23), followed by a 1,2-

Scheme 2.2

hydrogen shift in the formation of (2.25) and similar prototopic shifts in the conversion of (2.25) into fusicoccin (2.27) (Scheme 2.2). For this latter conversion two paths were, to start with, possible (a or b, Scheme 2.2). In the experiment that followed, [4-^{2}H$_2$, 3-^{13}C]mevalonic acid [as (2.22); labels in the same molecule] was found to give fusicoccin (2.27) in which the ^{13}C n.m.r. signals for C-7 and C-15 relative to the signals for C-11 and C-3 were markedly suppressed. This was attributable to C-7 and C-15 each having a deuterium attached (^{13}C has a longer relaxation time with deuterium attached than with hydrogen). There was also a small upfield shift of the signals for C-7 and C-15 consistent with ^{2}H attached to ^{13}C. Thus a deuterium atom was attached to each of C-7 and C-15, which, because of dilution of the label in the formation of (2.27), must have been derived from the *same* mevalonate molecule as the carbons to which they were attached. Thus the formation of (2.25) is as shown [a 1,3-shift from C-10 to quench the carbonium ion in (2.24) would also have given (2.27) with a deuterium and ^{13}C label on C-15 but they would have been from *different* mevalonate molecules; two adjacent mevalonate units were unlikely to be both labelled].

A deuterium atom at C-7 in (2.27) (and not C-3) as well as a ^{13}C label is consistent only with path a, Scheme 2.2, for the conversion of (2.25) into (2.27). [Path b and a 1,3-shift are again excluded, the latter by a similar argument to that employed in discussing the formation of (2.25) (Section 4.7)] [19].

Precursors with stable isotopic labels can provide further information not available with radioactive labels. Thus in the biosynthesis of microbial phenazines [as (2.29)], [2-^{2}H]shikimic acid (2.28) gave iodinin [as (2.29)] some molecules of which were dilabelled as

(2.28)   (2.29)

shown in (2.29) (measured by mass spectrometry). This proved that these symmetrical heterocycles are derived from two molecules of shikimic acid. Because of the symmetry in the metabolite, and the normal low enrichment of radioactive labels, ^{14}C and ^{3}H labels would not have allowed distinction between one and two molecules of precursor. The labelling sites, and thus orientation of (2.28) in (2.29), were established by base-catalysed exchange but, in principle, could have been determined by ^{2}H n.m.r. spectroscopy (Section 7.5.5).

2.3   Enzymes and mutants

Powerful support for any biosynthetic pathway as well as detailed information on the reactions involved may be gained by isolation, purification and characterization of enzymes which will catalyse individual steps of biosynthesis. A number of examples are quoted in succeeding chapters. The most notable are associated with the polyketide synthetases (Section 3.2) and enzymes of steroid biosynthesis (Sections 4.2 and 4.4).

An enzyme does not have to be pure to yield valuable information. In many cases simple cell-free preparations containing a mixture of many enzymes may yield most useful results. These preparations are simply made from bacterial cultures in various ways including ultrasonic disruption. For plants resort is commonly made to cell-free preparations from plant tissue cultures [20]. An impressive example is found in recent work on the biosynthesis of terpenoid indole alkaloids (Section 6.6.2). Also to be noted is the application here of radioimmunoassay [21] to the analysis of radioactive alkaloids.

A biosynthetic sequence can be summarized as A → B → C → D, where D is a known metabolite which is normally accumulated by the organism and A, B, and C are unknown intermediates. If the conversion of, e.g., B into C can be prevented through the absence of the necessary enzyme then B will accumulate instead of D. B may be isolated from this blocked, or mutant, organism and its structure determined. A second mutant may be blocked between C and D, so

C accumulates and may be identified.

In summary: mutant 1: A → B ⇸C → D
                        B accumulates
             mutant 2: A → B → C ⇸D
                        C accumulates.

If C is fed to mutant 1 then D will be produced. If B is fed to mutant 2, C will be produced. From this very simple example it can be concluded with reasonable security that the biosynthetic sequence to D involves B → C → D. In practice the situation is more complex. For applications in secondary metabolism see Section 3.8 and [2].

References

Further reading: [2]–[7].

[1] Robinson, R. (1955), *The Structural Relations of Natural Products*, Oxford University Press, Oxford.

[2] Brown, S. A. (1972), in *Biosynthesis* (*Specialist Periodical Reports*) (ed. T. A. Geissman), The Chemical Society, London, vol. 1, pp. 1–40.

[3] Simpson, T. J. (1975), *Chem. Soc. Rev.*, **4**, 497–522.

[4] Tanabe, M. (1973), in *Biosynthesis* (*Specialist Periodical Reports*) (ed. T. A. Geissman), The Chemical Society, London, vol. 2, pp. 241–99.

[5] Tanabe, M. (1975), in *Biosynthesis* (*Specialist Periodical Reports*) (ed. T. A. Geissman), The Chemical Society, vol. 3, pp. 247–85.

[6] Tanabe, M. (1976), in *Biosynthesis* (*Specialist Periodical Reports*) (ed. J. D. Bu'Lock), The Chemical Society, London, vol. 4, pp. 204–47.

[7] Garson, M. J. and Staunton, J. (1979), *Chem. Soc. Rev.*, **8**, 539–61.

[8] e.g. Murray, III, A. and Williams, D. L. (1958), *Organic Syntheses with Isotopes*, Interscience, New York, 2 vols.

[9] e.g. Leete, E. (1977), *J. Amer. Chem. Soc.*, **99**, 648–50.

[10] Battersby, A. R., Sheldrake, P. W. and Milner, J. A. (1974), *Tetrahedron Letters*, 3315–8.

[11] Gudgeon, J. A., Holker, J. S. E. and Simpson, T. J. (1974), *J. Chem. Soc. Chem. Comm.*, 636–8.

[12] Casey, M. L., Paulick, R. C. and Whitlock, jun., H. W. (1976), *J. Amer. Chem. Soc.*, **98**, 2636–40.

[13] Battersby, A. R., Fookes, C. J. R., McDonald, E. and Meegan, M. J. (1978), *J. Chem. Soc. Chem. Comm.*, 185–6.

[14] Battersby, A. R. and McDonald, E. (1979), *Acc. Chem. Res.*, **12**, 14–22 (review of porphyrin biosynthesis).

[15] Burton, G., Nordlöv, H., Hosozawa, S., Matsumoto, H., Jordan, P. M., Fagerness, P. E., Pryde, L. M. and Scott, A. I. (1979), *J. Amer. Chem. Soc.*, **101**, 3114–6.

[16] Booth, H., Bycroft, B. W., Wels, C. M., Corbett, K. and Maloney, A. P. (1976), *J. Chem. Soc. Chem. Comm.*, 110–1.

[17] Kainosho, M. (1979), *J. Amer. Chem. Soc.*, **101**, 1031–2 (for a cautionary note on the use of ^{15}N–^{13}C coupling).

[18] Popjak, G. and Cornforth, J. W. (1966), *Biochem. J.*, **101**, 553–68.

[19] Banerji, A., Hunter, R., Mellows, G., Sim, K. and Barton, D. H. R. (1978), *J. Chem. Soc. Chem. Comm.*, 843–5.
[20] Butcher, D. N. and Ingram, D. S. (1976), *Plant Tissue Culture*, Arnold, London.
[21] Chapman, D. I. (1979), *Chem. in Brit.*, **15**, 439–47.

3. Polyketides

3.1 Introduction

Acetic acid is found in living systems as its coenzyme A ester(*3.1*). This is a reactive thioester and is a pivotal compound in biosynthesis. On the one hand, it is involved in the formation of the important long-chain fatty acids and their transformation products (Section 1.1.2). On the other hand, (*3.1*) is the source of small fragments

(*3.1*) Acetyl ┊ coenzyme A

in the biosynthesis of numerous secondary metabolites whose origins chiefly lie elsewhere. There is, though, a large group of metabolites whose structures are legion [5] which is simply based, like the fatty acids, on the almost exclusive use of linear chains of repeating acetate units, generically the polyketides. This group of metabolites is the subject of discussion in this chapter but examples are to be found too in Chapters 5, 6 and 7. It should also be noted that the terpenes and steroids formed by repeating C_5 isoprene units derive ultimately from acetyl-coenzyme A (*3.1*) (Chapter 4). It seems that, in nature, little opportunity has been missed to use acetyl-coenzyme A to construct the backbone of many secondary metabolites or to embellish metabolites formed principally from other sources.

For those engaged in the structure determination of natural products there is a security to be found in structures which can be correlated with simple repeating units. So the repeating isoprene unit found in the terpenes (Chapter 4) has been invaluable in structure assignment. At the turn of the century Collie [6, 7] recognized that many natural products contained within them the $[CH_2\text{-}CO]_n$ unit and that this could be exploited in chemical synthesis, as in the conversion of dehydroacetic acid (*3.2*) via (*3.3*) into orsellinic acid (*3.4*),

Scheme 3.1

a naturally occurring polyketide. These ideas lay dormant until the middle of this century when Birch independently hypothesized that the biosynthesis of numerous secondary metabolites could be correlated with repeating CH_2-CO units based on acetate [8, 9]. Thus orsellinic acid *(3.4)* can be thought of as arising through the poly-β-keto-acyl-CoA derivative *(3.5)* [and not *(3.3)* which has an irregular $[CH_2$-CO$]_n$ sequence] derived by linear combination of acetate units (Scheme 3.2). The same triketo-intermediate *(3.5)* could lead to a

Scheme 3.2

number of other C_8 metabolites. Detailed discussion of the biosynthesis of these compounds is taken up in Section 3.3. It may be noted at this point though that the appropriate [1-^{14}C]acetate labelling of *(3.4)* (Scheme 3.2) and many other metabolites has been observed, thus validating the hypothesis [1].

Comparison of the illustrated pathway to *(3.5)* (Scheme 3.2; cf. Scheme 3.4) with that of fatty acid biosynthesis (Section 1.1.2; Scheme 1.2) indicates that a clear distinction between them is achieved by the absence of a reductase in polyketide formation, i.e. oxygen atoms of acetate are retained in polyketide metabolites. In the case of orsellinic acid *(3.4)*, in particular, results of experiments with [^{18}O]acetate established this to be correct [10]. It should be noted, however, that universal retention of acetate oxygen through the poly-β-keto-acyl-CoA to the final metabolite is not observed. One is missing, for example, in 6-methylsalicyclic acid *(3.14)* and several in curvularin *(3.87)*. (See, especially, Section 3.9 for what appear to be polyketides formed with varying levels of oxidation and dehydration corresponding to the steps illustrated in Scheme 1.2, Section 1.1.2.)

The Birch hypothesis initiated many studies on polyketide biosynthesis using [^{14}C]acetate, studies which have recently been extended in the impressive and powerful use of $[^{13}C]$acetate [11]. A second important consequence of the hypothesis has been in structure determination of natural products, thus returning to the original ideas of Collie. For example, at an early stage, the hypothesis indicated (correctly) that the structure of eleutherinol is (3.7) rather than (3.6) as originally thought [(3.7) may arise simply from the poly-β-keto-acyl-CoA (3.8); derivation of (3.6) would be more complex].

(3.6)   (3.7)   (3.8)

3.2   Formation of poly-β-keto-acyl-CoA's

3.2.1   Acetate and malonate [2, 12, 13]

Formation of a poly-β-keto-acyl-CoA [as (3.9)] occurs as for fatty acid biosynthesis by condensation of acetyl-coenzyme A with malonyl-CoA. Malonyl-CoA is generally derived by carboxylation of (3.1) (Scheme 3.3). An alternative path to malonyl-CoA is via oxaloacetate, an intermediate in the citric acid cycle.

Scheme 3.3   (3.9) Poly-β-ketoacyl-CoA

Incorporation of $[1\text{-}^{14}C]$acetate into a polyketide metabolite gives labelling throughout the chain, of alternate carbon atoms, which are of course the normally oxygenated ones. Labelled malonate, on the other hand, tends to label the second and successive acetate-derived units more heavily than the first [*unit in (3.9)] which derives directly from acetate and not malonate. This first acetate unit is called 'starter' acetate.

Assimilation of $[1\text{-}^{14}C]$acetate into an organism may be followed by direct conversion into a polyketide metabolite, or the labelled acid may be turned through the citric acid cycle before use in polyketide biosynthesis. The result is, however, that $[1\text{-}^{14}C]$acetate is again generated. On the other hand, $[2\text{-}^{14}C]$acetate which enters the citric acid cycle exits with some label on C-1 in addition to that on C-2. Thus, $[2\text{-}^{14}\text{C}]$acetate can lead to a polyketide with label distributed over all its carbon atoms.

Some polyketides include extra carbon atoms as $[\text{CHRCO}]_n$, $R = H$ and Me. The extra C_1 units may arise from S-adenosylmethionine with methylation of an intermediate enol [as $(3.22) \rightarrow (3.23)$]. Alternatively introduction is by substitution in biosynthesis of propionyl-CoA (3.10) and methylmalonyl-CoA (3.11) for, respectively, acetyl-CoA and malonyl-CoA. Although (3.11) may derive by carboxylation of (3.10) as for the lower homologues, it is believed that normal biosynthesis is the reverse: (3.10) is formed by decarboxylation of methylmalonyl-CoA (3.11). This compound,

$$\text{CH}_3\text{-CH}_2\text{-C-S-CoA} \qquad \text{CH}_3\text{-CH-C-S-CoA}$$

(3.10) Propionyl-CoA   *(3.11)* Methylmalonyl-CoA

(3.11), is derived from the citric acid-cycle intermediate, succinyl-CoA in a B_{12} mediated reaction. For examples on the utilization of (3.10) and (3.11) in biosynthesis see Sections 3.8, 3.9 and 7.6.1. The use of a malonamyl residue [see (3.97)] as a starter unit in tetracycline biosynthesis (Section 3.8) is to be noted as is the important one of cinnamoyl-CoA in flavone biosynthesis (Section 5.4).

3.2.2 Assembly of poly-β-keto-acyl-CoA's

Formation of a polyketide involves condensation of acetyl-CoA with the appropriate number of malonyl-CoA units, modification of the completed poly-β-ketone where required, and release of the product in stable form, as, for example, in 6-methylsalicylic acid biosynthesis (Scheme 3.4). The whole sequence occurs enzyme-bound, without release, or acceptance, of intermediates externally. Thus probing of the biosynthetic sequence by normal feeding experiments with possible intermediates fails. Instead, very properly, information is gained in different ways by working with the actual enzymes involved. The biosynthesis of several polyketides has been explored in this way, and most extensively that of 6-methylsalicyclic acid (3.14) [14–17].

Extensive purification of 6-methylsalicylate synthetase from *Penicillium patulum* has been carried out. It is distinct from fatty acid synthetase, separable from it, and of half the molecular weight; both enzymes are complexes of several enzymes. One molecule of 6-methylsalicylic acid is generated by 6-methylsalicylate synthetase from one molecule of acetyl-CoA and three of malonyl-CoA in the presence of one molecule of NADPH as coenzyme; no free intermediates can be detected. In the absence of NADPH, triacetic acid lactone (3.15) is formed as the sole product. The same lactone is

Scheme 3.4

formed when coenzyme is omitted from reactions of fatty acid synthetases derived from a variety of sources. So there are similarities in the way the two enzymes function. There are differences, however. Most obviously in 6-methylsalicylate formation reduction occurs only once (with eventual formation of a *cis*-double bond) and at a late stage, whereas for fatty acids reduction occurs after each malonate addition (cf. Scheme 1.2; Section 1.1.2). Also, it has been observed that the rate of (*3.15*) formation is higher with 6-methylsalicylate synthetase than with fatty acid synthetase, both isolated from *P. patulum*.

The similarities in the function of the two enzymes and of course in the substrates has suggested that the mechanisms of enzyme action are similar. Also, the 6-methylsalicylate synthetase has two different types of thiol grouping (deduced from inhibition studies) which are analogous to the ACP carrier and condensing sites in fatty acid synthetase. A possible mechanism of (*3.14*) formation is illustrated in Scheme 3.4. The different receptors for the malonate electron pair through the sequence contrasts with a uniformity of receptor type in fatty acid biosynthesis (see Scheme 1.2, Section 1.1.2). The *cis*-double bond in (*3.13*) can be thought of as conferring on the growing chain the requisite conformation for eventual cyclization. Where reduction does not occur, as in orsellinic acid (*3.4*) synthesis, conformational rigidity can be achieved via the enol forms of the keto-groups. In some cases *C*-methyl groups may also affect the conformation of the folded chain (Section 3.9).

C-Methylation occurs before release of the completed polyketide from the synthetase complex. The evidence for this conclusion comes in part from the failure of unmethylated compounds to serve as precursors, e.g. orsellenic acid (*3.4*) is not a precursor for atranorin (*3.16*) [18]. Similarly 5-methylorcylaldehyde (*3.18*), and not orcyldehyde (*3.17*), is a precursor for gliorosein (*3.19*) and related compounds [19]. Barnol (*3.20*) is interesting in that one methyl group

(3.15)   (3.16) Atranorin   (3.17) R=H   (3.19) Gliorosein   (3.20) Barnol
                            (3.18) R=Me

derives from methionine (*) and the other by reduction of a carboxy-group. The ethyl group derives from C-2 of acetate and methionine. [The polyketide skeleton, as (*3.5*), is revealed by the dotted lines in (*3.20*)] [20].

Incorporation of [^{2}H$_3$]methionine into gliorosein (*3.19*) occurs with retention of all the deuterium atoms [21] arguing for methylation by a simple nucleophilic displacement on *S*-adenosylmethionine [see (*3.22*)].

Aspergillus flaviceps normally produces 5-methylorsellinic acid| (*3.24*) and its transformation product flavipin (*3.25*). A cell-free enzyme preparation used [^{14}CH$_3$]methionine for formation of the aromatic metabolite [in this case, 5,6-dimethylresorcinol, as (*3.24*)] without addition of any poly-β-keto-acyl-CoA acceptor. So this substrate was already enzyme bound. Various products derivable from (*3.21*) were obtained on hydrolysis of the enzyme complex thus indicating (*3.21*) to be the substrate for methylation (Scheme 3.5) [22]. This is a second piece of evidence for methylation occurring before release of the completed polyketide from the synthetase complex.

1 x Acetyl - CoA
+ 3 x Malonyl - CoA

(3.21)   S-Adenosyl methionine

(3.22)

(3.23)   S-Enz

(3.25) Flavipin   (3.24) 5-Methylorsellinic acid

Scheme 3.5

Prenylation in contrast to methylation occurs on the polyketide after liberation from the enzyme (see mycophenolic acid, Section 4.6). A normal prenylation occurs here, and in the formation of (3.26), *ortho* to a phenolic hydroxy-group, see Scheme 3.6; siccanin (3.27) derives from (3.26) [23].

Scheme 3.6

Commonly for polyketides, $n = 4$ to 10 in the general formulation $[CH_2\text{-}CO]_n$ but may be as high as 19 to 20 in macrolide antibiotics (Sections 3.9 and 7.6.1). Numerous examples are known where $n = 4, 5, 7$ and 8 while those where $n = 3, 6, 9$ and 10 are less common. Cyclization of a poly-β-keto-acyl-CoA chain to give a six-membered ring can take a number of courses. Almost all the possible cyclization modes are represented in naturally occurring polyketides with, apparently, a single restriction. Uncyclized residues from the methyl end of a polyketide are never shorter than the residues bearing the carboxy group. Thus cyclization of (3.28) may occur as shown but not as in (3.29). This clearly relates in some (unknown)

(3.28)   (3.29)

way to the mechanism of ring closure. It is also observed that whatever oxygens are deleted in a polyketide the one next to a carboxy group as in (3.14), is always retained. It may be concluded that the anion (enol) used in cyclization α to a thioester function requires stabilization by both the ketonic and thioester carbonyl group.

3.3   Tetraketides

The biosynthesis of some examples of this numerous group of polyketides is summarized in Scheme 3.7. Note: (i) the single and particular labelling site in fumigatin (3.33) derived from orsellinic acid indicates the orientation of the original poly-β-keto-acyl-CoA. Also that the carboxy-group is lost after introduction of the C-5 hydroxy-group; otherwise a symmetrical intermediate [(3.40); labelling as shown] and dilabelled (3.33) would have been generated; (ii) the formation of usnic acid (3.37) is by oxidative coupling (Section 1.3.1)

Scheme 3.7

of two molecules of methylphloroacetophenone (*3.36*). Further examples in tetraketide biosynthesis are (*3.14*), (*3.16*), (*3.19*), (*3.20*), (*3.25*), and (*3.27*); see below also.

Tetraketides are formed from four acetate/malonate units. This is the minimum number for formation of a common stable aromatic ring. As already seen, *inter alia*, in orsellinic acid (*3.4*) the oxygenation pattern is an alternatimg one. Aromatic rings formed from phenylalanine and tyrosine (Chapter 5) have a different pattern, as seen in (*3.41*). [A particularly good example, where one aromatic ring derives from acetate/malonate and a second from phenylalanine, is found in the flavonoids (Section 5.4).] At its simplest then one can distinguish visually between these two alternative routes to aromatic rings. Further aromatic oxygenation of course blurs the visual distinction, see *(3.20)*, as does the loss of polyketide oxygen during biosynthesis.

The biosynthesis of the aromatic metabolite, 6-methylsalicylic acid *(3.14)*, has been discussed above. This acid is the source of a variety of metabolites in which hydroxylation and oxidation of the aromatic nucleus and side-chain methyl group occur in major pathways [4] following decarboxylation to *m*-cresol *(3.42)*. A terminus in this set of oxidative reactions is patulin *(3.45)*.

Scheme 3.8

The [1-^{14}C]acetate labelling in patulin is shown (●). No regular polyketide chain is apparent but the incorporation of radioactive 6-methylsalicylic acid *(3.14)* and other related compounds indicate that *(3.45)* arises by cleavage of an aromatic ring [see dotted line in *(3.44)*].

An interesting experiment [32] relates to the incorporation of *m*-[^{2}H$_{3}$]cresol *(3.46)*. Dideuteriopatulin was isolated, the mass spectral fragmentation of which was consistent with location of deuterium as in *(3.47)*, and the cleavage as in Scheme 3.8.

Enzyme preparations from *P. patulum* have been obtained which have been studied for their substrate specificity and products formed. For example, one preparation converted *m*-hydroxybenzyl alcohol *(3.43)* into gentisyl alcohol *(3.38)* but the corresponding aldehyde *(3.48)* was not ring-hydroxylated by any preparation from *P. patulum*. Thus *(3.43)* but not *(3.48)* is on the pathway to patulin *(3.45)*. All the various strands of evidence [32, 33] lead to the pathway shown in Scheme 3.8.

A different cleavage of an aromatic ring is apparent in penicillic acid *(3.31)* formation. Penicillic acid has its genesis via orsellinic acid

(3.49), and labelling of (3.31) = (3.50) by [1,2-$^{13}C_2$]acetate, see (3.49) → (3.50), allows clear definition of the site of aromatic ring

cleavage as that shown [dotted line in (3.30) and (3.49)]. Results of precursor feeding experiments indicate the sequence of biosynthesis which is abbreviated in Scheme 3.7. An enzyme preparation which effects the final oxidative ring opening has been isolated; it is a mono-oxygenase [24–26]. Similar enzymes, working on quinones [see (3.30)] as substrates for aromatic ring opening, may be involved in the biosynthesis of patulin (3.45), also multicolic acid and the aflatoxins (which are discussed below).

A mono-oxygenase is also implicated in the biosynthesis of fungal tropolones, e.g. stipitatonic acid (3.52). Ring expansion of an aromatic ring could, as in colchicine biosynthesis, account for the formation of the tropolone ring (Section 6.3.7). This is strongly supported by the appropriate specific incorporation of labelled 3-methylorsellinic acid (3.51) into stipitatonic acid (3.52), and $^{18}O_2$

labelling results [see (3.52)] [34, 35]. Another tropolone-containing metabolite, sepedonin (3.54), derives from a pentaketide with inclusion of a C_1 unit [*site in (3.54)]. By analogy with stipitatonic acid biosynthesis (3.53) is a likely intermediate [36, 37].

(3.53)   (3.54) Sepedonin

(3.55) Colletodiol

† Colletodiol (3.55) is a simple non-aromatic polyketide. [^{13}C]Acetate labelling is consistent with its formation by union of a tetraketide with a triketide formalized as shown [38].

3.4 Pentaketides

Pentaketides are formed from five acetate/malonate units. Commonly compounds of type (3.53) are produced which are further modified as for the tetraketides in ways which include aromatic ring scission. A simple modification is in the formation of isocoumarins [as (3.58)]. Citrinin (3.57) is believed to be derived via (3.56) [39].

(3.56)   (3.57) Citrinin

† The isocoumarin (3.58) is produced along with terrein (3.59) by some strains of *Aspergillus terreus*; and (3.58) is a precursor for (3.59). Results of experiments with [$^{13}C_2$]acetate indicate that formation of (3.59) occurs by fracture of (3.58) in the manner shown (Scheme 3.9, path a; thickened bonds: intact acetate units) [40]. A compound, (3.60), with related structure is thought to be formed in a slightly different manner (Scheme 3.9, path b) [41]. A third variation on the

(3.58)   (3.59) Terrein

(3.60)

Scheme 3.9

fragmentation theme, (3.61) → (3.62), has again been deduced from [$^{13}C_2$]acetate labelling [42].

(3.61)   (3.62)

† The pattern of [^{13}C]-acetate and -methionine incorporation in sclerin (3.64) indicates biosynthesis from *two* polyketide chains, as (3.63). An alternative attractive suggestion is that (3.64) has its genesis in a precursor with a single polyketide chain [as (3.65)] through an isocoumarin co-metabolite, sclerotinin A (3.66) (Scheme 3.10) [43, 44].

† [2-^{13}C]Acetate labelling [● in (3.67)] of asperlin (3.67) indicates a simple unfragmented polyketide chain [45].

(3.63)   (3.64) Sclerin

(3.65)   (3.66)

Scheme 3.10

(3.67) Asperlin

3.5 Hexaketides

† Relatively few hexaketides have been isolated. Variotin (3.68) is an example. It derives in the expected manner from acetate (malonate) and methionine with the pyrrolidone ring having its origins in glutamic acid [46, 47]. Labelled acetate and formate (source via methionine for methyl groups) were incorporated into alternaric acid (3.69) in a manner consistent with condensation of a hexaketide-derived acyl derivative with dihydrotriacetic acid lactone [see dotted line in (3.69)] [48]. Rubropunctatin (3.70) can be split into two

(3.68) Variotin

(3.69) Alternaric acid

(3.70) Rubropunctatin

fragments on the basis of labelling results (dotted line). The right-hand part derives in the usual way; the left-hand part though seems to derive through the β-keto acid formed by condensation of hexanoic acid with an acetate unit [49, 50].

† Multicolic acid (3.72) is a fragmented polyketide. $[^{13}C_2]$Acetate gave results which indicate the manner of biosynthesis as that shown in Scheme 3.11. The arrangement shown requires C-4,5 cleavage before loss of the carboxy-group. Otherwise the symmetrical intermediate (3.73) would be involved with consequent alteration of the

1 x Acetate
5 x Malonate

(3.71)

(3.72) Multicolic acid

(3.73)

Scheme 3.11

^{13}C labelling pattern arising from C-4,5 and equivalent C-1,2 cleavage [51].

3.6 Heptaketides

Proof that griseofulvin (3.76) is formed by linear combination of acetate units provided early key support for Birch's polyketide hypothesis. The benzophenone (3.75) is a likely intermediate. It can give griseofulvin by oxidative coupling (see Section 1.3.1) followed by saturation of one of the double-bonds in the resultant dienone. [2-^{3}H$_3$]Acetate labelled the positions indicated in (3.76) in accord with ^{14}C data and the pathway shown (Scheme 3.12). Moreover, the

(3.74)

(3.75)

Scheme 3.12

(3.76) Griseofulvin

results show that double-bond saturation in the intermediate dienone involves *trans* addition of hydrogen [52, 53].

† As the poly-β-keto-acyl-CoA chain gets longer so the opportunity increases for widely differing cyclization reactions. A minor variation on the pattern in griseofulvin is seen in alternariol (3.77) formation from a single chain [54]. A quite different pattern is found in the

(3.77) Alternariol

(3.78) Deoxyherquienone

(3.79) Cercosporin

fungal phenalenones, e.g. deoxyherquienone (*3.78*) (see dotted lines) [55]. Interestingly the plant phenalenones derive from phenylalanine, tyrosine and a single acetate (malonate) [56, 57].

† Increasing complexity is seen in metabolites like cercosporin (*3.79*) which is formed by oxidative coupling of two heptaketide units [58].

3.7 Octaketides

A common structural type is that of an anthraquinone, e.g. islandicin (*3.80*). Ring cleavage leads on, for example, to xanthones, e.g. ravenilin (*3.82*). The pattern of islandicin biosynthesis is indicated in Scheme 3.13 [59]. Islandicin (*3.80*) is plausibly an intermediate in

(3.80) Islandicin

(3.81)

(3.82) Ravenilin

Scheme 3.13

ravenilin (*3.82*) biosynthesis; the [$^{13}C_2$]acetate labelling pattern is consistent with this possibility. (The labelling pattern is a mixture of two arising plausibly as shown in Scheme 3.13 [60].) The biosynthesis of sulochrin (*3.84*) has been proven to be analogously via the anthraquinone (*3.83*), derived in turn from acetate/malonate [61].

† Study of mollisin (*3.85*) biosynthesis provides a particularly good

(3.83)

(3.84) Sulochrin

(3.85) Mollisin

Scheme 3.14

example where $[^{13}C_2]$acetate has cleared up uncertainties in biosynthesis arising from ^{14}C labelling data. The results are that the naphthoquinone (*3.85*) is formed as shown (Scheme 3.14) either via a simple fragmented octaketide chain or two separate chains [62]. (For further discussion of quinone biosynthesis see Section 5.2.)

† Brefeldin (*3.86*) is a quite different octaketide. It derives again by simple linear combination of eight acetate/malonate units [63] as does curvularin (*3.87*) [64]. Ochrephilone (*3.88*) biosynthesis on the

(*3.86*) Brefeldin

(*3.87*) Curvularin

(*3.88*) Ochrephilone

other hand is more complex. This metabolite appears to originate from two polyketide chains with inclusion of three *C*-methyl groups (see dotted lines) [65].

3.8 Nona- and deca-ketides

Bikaverin (*3.89*) is a rare example of a nonaketide. It is formed by simple folding of a single chain (see dotted line) [66].

(*3.89*) Bikaverin

The aflatoxins, e.g. aflatoxin B_1 (*3.95*), are an important group of toxins. They have provided a significant investigative challenge because they are such severely modified polyketides. There has also been some recent confusion because of misassignment of ^{13}C n.m.r. resonances. However, the same pattern of biosynthesis is now clear for the aflatoxins and for sterigmatocystin (*3.93*) which is a highly efficient aflatoxin precursor. The structures, particularly of metabolites produced by mutants and established conversions, together with the ^{13}C labelling data, allow an outline pathway to sterigmatocystin (*3.93*) through to aflatoxins B_1 (*3.95*) and G_1 (*3.96*) to be deduced (Scheme 3.15) [4, 67–72]. Averufin (*3.92*) is an early intermediate in this pathway. Detection of ^{18}O label by ^{18}O-induced shifts in the ^{13}C n.m.r. spectrum of (*3.92*) derived from $^{18}O_2$ and from $[1-^{13}C, ^{18}O_2]$acetate has allowed precise confirmation of the level of oxygenation in the early stages of the biosynthetic pathway in Scheme 3.15. (Incidental powerful confirmation of retention of acetate oxygen atoms into polyketides in general is also provided by this decaketide example [73].)

(3.90) (3.91) (3.92) Averufin

(3.93) Sterigmatocystin

(3.96) Aflatoxin G₁

(3.95) Aflatoxin B₁

(3.94)

Scheme 3.15

Tetracyclines, e.g. 7-chlorotetracycline (*3.100*), are commercially important broad-spectrum antibiotics. Detailed information is available on the course of their biosynthesis as a result of an extensive study, using mutants in particular. This involved isolation of new products from differently blocked mutants and testing them as precursors in cross-feeding experiments. The structure (*3.99*) of mutant produced protetrone indicates the manner of folding in the polyketide as (*3.97*) (protetrone is a diversion from the main path-

(3.97)

(3.98)

(3.99)

(3.100) 7-Chlorotetracycline

Scheme 3.16

way, however). This polyketide is notable for its malonamyl starter [see (*3.97*)].

The deduced sequence to 7-chlorotetracycline (*3.100*) is illustrated in brief in Scheme 3.16. As commonly for polyketides, methylation occurs at the enzyme-bound stage on (*3.97*). Chlorination occurs on an aromatic ring (electrophilic substitution by Cl^+ on an electron-rich aromatic nucleus).

† A different mode of poly-β-ketone folding to that of the tetracyclines is observed for the anthracycline glycosidic antibiotics. ε-Pyrromycinone (*3.101*), an example of the aglycone fragment in

(3.101) ε -Pyrromycinone

these antibiotics, is derived from nine acetate units as shown by the dotted line; the chain starter is propionate [75].

3.9   Polyketides with mixed origins

The very largest of the polyketides are the macrolide antibiotics, e.g. nystatin (*3.106*). Further examples are the ansamycins which derive by a mixed acetate–propionate pathway (Section 7.6.1). Intermediate in size are the cytochalasins which derive by an acetate (malonate) pathway (Section 7.6.2). Where propionate units account for C_3 fragments in the ansamycins, methionine and acetate serve in the cytochalasins. The macrolide antibiotics discussed below all follow the former way of generating C_3 units. It is clear that, if methyl groups are introduced by two different pathways, this is not adventitious. The methyl groups must have a function possibly like the double bonds in dictating the conformation of the macrocycle.

For the biosynthesis of these complex polyketides, ^{13}C labelled precursors have been used to great advantage in plotting the origins of macrocyclic antibiotics. Little is known, however, of the mechanism of biosynthesis. (For a discussion on the possible significance of templates see [4].)

Tylosin (*3.102*) is formed as indicated, the one C_4 unit deriving from ethylmalonate (= butyrate) [76]. A similar origin is apparent for leucomycin (*3.103*) but the origin of C-3 and C-4 is obscure (not labelled by $[1-^{13}C]$-, $[2-^{13}C]$-acetate, $[1-^{13}C]$propionate or $[1-^{13}C]$butyrate) [77]. In both studies extensive catabolism of butyrate and ethylmalonate into propionyl fragments was observed, but by different pathways.

† The platenomycins are closely related to leucomycin [78]. Picromycin (*3.104*) has its genesis from six propionate units and one

(3.102) Tylosin

$\bullet\!\!-\!\!\bullet$ = CH_3CO_2H

$\frown\!\!\bullet$ = $CH_3CH_2CO_2H$

$\vee\!\!\!-\!\!\bullet$ = $CH_3CH_2CH_2CO_2H$

(3.103) Leucomycin

(3.104) Picromycin

(3.105) Erythromycin A

(3.106) Nystatin

acetate [80]. Erythromycin A (3.105) is wholly derived from propionate [81, 82]. Sixteen acetate and three propionate units account for the skeleton of the aglycone unit of nystatin (3.106) [83].

† Mixed origins have been deduced for aureothin (3.107) from propionate and (probably) a single acetate plus p-nitrobenzoic acid [84], and for (3.108) which derives from acetate, propionate, and butyrate [85]. Avenaciolide (3.109) derives from acetate/malonate plus

(3.107)

(3.108)

1 x Acetyl-CoA
5 x Malonyl-CoA $\Big\}$ ⟶

$CH_2 - CH_2CO_2H$

(3.109) Avenaciolide

Scheme 3.17

succinyl-CoA (Scheme 3.17). Label from both [1-^{13}C]- and [2-^{13}C]-acetate is transferred to succinyl-CoA through the citric acid cycle. [The avenaciolide was labelled directly then by acetate and indirectly through succinate.] In (3.109) derived from [2-^{13}C]acetate coupling was observed between C-11 and C-15 in the ^{13}C n.m.r. spectrum consonant with a succinate origin for C-15, C-11 and C-12. (At a high enough ^{13}C concentration two C-2-labelled acetate units will join together to give succinyl-CoA with two continuous ^{13}C labels [86].)

References

Further reading: [1]–[4]; *Biosynthesis (Specialist Periodical Reports)* [ed. T. A. Geissman (vols. 1–3), J. D. Bu'Lock (vols. 4 and 5)], The Chemical Society, London.

[1] Turner, W. B. (1971), *Fungal Metabolites*, Academic Press, London.
[2] Packter, N. M. (1973), *Biosynthesis of Acetate-derived Compounds*, Wiley, London.
[3] Packter, N. M. (1980), in *The Biochemistry of Plants* (ed. P. K. Stumpf), Academic Press, London, vol. 4, pp. 535–70 (I am grateful to Dr Packter for the opportunity to read his manuscript before publication).
[4] Bu'Lock, J. D. (1979), in *Comprehensive Organic Chemistry* (eds. D. H. R. Barton and W. D. Ollis), Pergamon, Oxford, vol. 5, pp. 927–87.
[5] cf. *St. Mark's Gospel*, chapter 5, vv. 9–13.
[6] Collie, J. N. (1907), *J. Chem. Soc.*, **91**, 1806–13.
[7] Stewart, A. W. and Graham, H. (1948), *Recent Advances in Organic Chemistry*, 7th edn., Longmans, Green and Co., London, vol. 2, ch. 13.
[8] Birch, A. J. and Donovan, F. W. (1953), *Aust. J. Chem.*, **6**, 360–8.
[9] Birch, A. J. (1957), *Fortschritte der Chemie Organischer Naturstoffe*, **14**, 186–216; (1962), *Proc. Chem. Soc.*, 3–13.
[10] Gatenbeck, S. and Mosbach, K. (1959), *Acta Chem. Scand.*, **12**, 1561–4.
[11] Simpson, T. J. (1975), *Chem. Soc. Rev.*, **4**, 497–522.
[12] Mahler, H. R. and Cordes, E. H. (1971), *Biological Chemistry*, 2nd Edn, Harper and Row, New York.
[13] Spenser, I. D. (1968), in *Comprehensive Biochemistry* (eds. M. Florkin and E. H. Stotz), Elsevier, Amsterdam, vol. 20, p. 231–413 (for acetate labelling via the tricarboxylic acid cycle).
[14] Dimroth, P., Ringelmann, E. and Lynen, F. (1976), *Eur. J. Biochem.*, **68**, 591–6.
[15] Scott, A. I., Beadling, L. C., Georgopapadakou, N. H. and Subbarayan, C. R. (1974), *Bio-org. Chem.*, **3**, 238–48.
[16] Light, R. J. and Hager, L. P. (1968), *Arch. Biochem. Biophys.*, **125**, 326–33.
[17] Vogel, G. and Lynen, F. (1975), *Methods Enzymol.*, **43**, 520–30.
[18] Yamazaki, M. and Shibata, S. (1966), *Chem. Pharm. Bull. (Japan)*, **14**, 96–7.
[19] Steward, M. W. and Packter, N. M. (1968), *Biochem. J.*, **109**, 1–11.
[20] Mosbach, K. and Ljungcrantz, I. (1965), *Physiol. Plantarum*, **18**, 1–7.
[21] Lenfant, M., Farrugia, G. and Lederer, M. (1969), *Compt. rend.*, **268D**, 1986–9.

[22] Gatenbeck, S., Eriksson, P. O. and Hansson, Y. (1969), *Acta Chem. Scand.*, **23**, 699–701.

[23] Suzuki, K. T. and Nozoe, S. (1974), *Bio-org. Chem.*, **3**, 72–80.

[24] Seto, H., Cary, L. W. and Tanabe, M. (1974), *J. Antibiotics*, **27**, 558–9.

[25] Axberg, K. and Gatenbeck, S. (1975), *Acta Chem. Scand.*, **B29**, 749–51.

[26] Axberg, K. and Gatenbeck, S. (1975), *FEBS Lett.*, **54**, 18–20.

[27] Bentley, R. (1965), in *Biogenesis of Antibiotic Substances* (ed. Z. Vanek and Z. Hostalek), Academic Press, New York, pp. 241–54.

[28] Petterson, G. (1965), *Acta Chem. Scand.*, **19**, 543–8; 1016–7.

[29] Gatenbeck, S. and Brunsberg, U. (1966), *Acta Chem. Scand.*, **20**, 2334–8.

[30] Taguchi, H., Sankawa, U. and Shibata, S. (1969), *Chem. Pharm. Bull. (Japan)*, **17**, 2054–60.

[31] Nabeta, K., Ichihara, A. and Sakamura, S. (1975), *Agric. Biol. Chem. (Japan)*, **39**, 409–13.

[32] Scott, A. I. and Yalpani, M. (1967), *Chem. Comm.*, 945–6.

[33] Murphy, G. and Lynen, F. (1975), *Eur. J. Biochem.*, **58**, 467–75.

[34] Scott, A. I. and Wiesner, K. J. (1972), *J. Chem. Soc. Chem. Comm.*, 1075–7.

[35] Scott, A. I. and Lee, E. (1972), *J. Chem. Soc. Chem. Comm.*, pp. 655–6.

[36] McInnes, A. G., Smith, D. G., Vining, L. C. and Johnson, L. (1971), *J. Chem. Soc. Chem. Comm.*, 325–6.

[37] Takenaka, S. and Seto, S. (1971), *Agric. Biol. Chem. (Japan)*, **35**, 862–9.

[38] Lunnon, M. W. and MacMillan, J. (1976), *J. Chem. Soc. Perkin I*, 184–6.

[39] Barber, J. and Staunton, J. (1979), *J. Chem. Soc. Chem. Comm.*, 1098–9.

[40] Hill, R. A., Carter, R. H. and Staunton, J. (1975), *J. Chem. Soc. Chem. Comm.*, 380–1.

[41] Holker, J. S. E. and Young, K. (1975), *J. Chem. Soc. Chem. Comm.*, 525–6.

[42] Simpson, T. J. and Holker, J. S. E. (1975), *Tetrahedron Lett.*, 4693–6.

[43] Cox, R. E. and Holker, J. S. E. (1976), *J. Chem. Soc. Perkin I*, 2077–9.

[44] Garson, M. J. and Staunton, J. (1976), *J. Chem. Soc. Chem. Comm.*, 928–9.

[45] Tanabe, M., Hamasaki, T., Thomas, D. and Johnson, L. (1971), *J. Amer. Chem. Soc.*, **93**, 273–4.

[46] Tanake, N. and Umezawa, H. (1962), *J. Antibiotics*, **15**, 189–9.

[47] Tanake, N., Sashikata, K. and Umezawa, H. (1962), *J. Antibiotics*, **15**, 228–9.

[48] Turner, W. B. (1961), *J. Chem. Soc.*, 522–4.

[49] Kurono, M., Nakanishi, K., Shindo, K. and Tada, M. (1963), *Chem. Pharm. Bull. (Japan)*, **11**, 359–62.

[50] Hadfield, J. R., Holker, J. S. E. and Stanway, D. N. (1967), *J. Chem. Soc. (C)*, 751–5.

[51] Gudgeon, J. A., Holker, J. S. E. and Simpson, T. J. (1974), *J. Chem. Soc. Chem. Comm.*, 636–8.

[52] Birch, A. J., Massy-Westropp, R. A., Richards, R. W. and Smith, H. (1958), *J. Chem. Soc.*, 360–5.

[53] Sato, Y., Machida, T. and Oda, T. (1975), *Tetrahedron Letters*, 4571–4.

[54] Sjöland, S. and Gatenbeck, S. (1966), *Acta Chem. Scand.*, **20**, 1053–9.

[55] Simpson, T. J. (1976), *J. Chem. Soc. Chem. Comm.*, 258–60.

[56] Thomas, R. (1971), *J. Chem. Soc. Chem. Comm.*, 739–40.

[57] Edwards, J. M., Schmitt, R. C. and Weiss, U. (1972), *Phytochemistry*, **11**, 1717–20.

[58] Okubo, A., Yamazaki, S. and Fuwa, K. (1975), *Agric. Biol. Chem. (Japan)*, **39**, 1173–5.

[59] Paulick, R. C., Casey, M. L., Hillenbrand, D. F. and Whitlock, H. W. jun., (1975), *J. Amer. Chem. Soc.*, **97**, 5303–5.

[60] Birch, A. J., Baldas, J., Hlubucek, R., Simpson, T. J. and Westerman, P. W. (1976), *J. Chem. Soc. Perkin I*, 898–904.

[61] Curtis, R. F., Hassall, C. H. and Parry, D. R. (1972), *J. Chem. Soc. Perkin I*, 240–4.

[62] Casey, M. L., Paulick, R. C. and Whitlock, H. W. jun., (1976), *J. Amer. Chem. Soc.*, **98**, 2636–40.

[63] Cross, B. E. and Hendley, P. (1975), *J. Chem. Soc. Chem. Comm.*, 124–5.

[64] Birch, A. J., Musgrave, O. C., Rickards, R. W. and Smith, H. (1959), *J. Chem. Soc. (C)*, 3146–52.

[65] Kamiya, Y., Ikegami, S. and Tamura, S. (1974), *Tetrahedron Lett.*, 655–8.

[66] McInnes, A. G., Smith, D. G., Walter, J. A., Vining, L. C. and Wright, J. L. C. (1975), *J. Chem. Soc. Chem. Comm.*, 66–8.

[67] Pachler, K. G. R., Steyn, P. S., Vleggaar, R., Wessels, P. L. and Scott, D. B. (1976), *J. Chem. Soc. Perkin I*, 1182–9.

[68] Elsworthy, G. C., Holker, J. S. E., McKeown, J. M., Robinson, J. B. and Mulheirn, L. J. (1970), *Chem. Comm.*, 1069–70.

[69] Heathcote, J. G., Dutton, M. F. and Hibbert, J. R. (1976), *Chem. Ind.*, (*London*) 270–2.

[70] Roberts, J. C. (1974), *Fortschritte der Chemie Organischer Naturstoffe*, **31**, 120–51.

[71] Zamir, L. O. and Ginsburg, R. (1979), *J. Bacteriol.*, **138**, 684–90.

[72] Singh, R. and Hsieh, D. P. (1977), *Arch. Biochem., Biophys.*, **178**, 285–92.

[73] Vederas, J. C. and Nakashima, T. T. (1980), *J. Chem. Soc. Chem. Comm.*, 183–5.

[74] McCormick, J. R. D. and Jensen, E. R. (1968), *J. Amer. Chem. Soc.*, **90**, 7126–7; and following paper.

[75] Ollis, W. D., Sutherland, I. O., Codner, R. C., Gordon, J. J. and Miller, G. A. (1960), *Proc. Chem. Soc.*, 347–9.

[76] Ōmura, S., Nakagawa, A., Takeshima, H., Miyazawa, J., Kitao, C., Piriou, F. and Lukacs, G. (1975), *Tetrahedron Lett.*, 4503–6.

[77] Ōmura, S., Nakagawa, A., Takeshima, H., Atusmi, K., Miyazawa, J., Piriou, F. and Lukacs, G. (1975), *J. Amer. Chem. Soc.*, **97**, 6600–2.

[78] Furumai, T. and Suzuki, M. (1975), *J. Antibiotics*, **28**, 770–4; 775–82; 783–8.

[79] Furumai, T., Takeda, K. and Suzuki, M. (1975), *J. Antibiotics*, **28**, 789–97.

[80] Ōmura, S., Takeshima, H., Nakagawa, A., Miyazawa, J. and Lukacs, G. (1975), *J. Antibiotics*, **29**, 316–7.

[81] Grisebach, H., Hofheinz, W. and Achenbach, H. (1962), *Z. Naturforsch.*, **17b**, 64–5.

[82] Martin, J. R., Egan, R. S., Goldstein, A. W. and Collum, P. (1975), *Tetrahedron*, **31**, 1985–9.

[83] Birch, A. J., Holzapfel, C. W., Rickards, R. W., Djerassi, C., Suzuki, M., Westley, J., Dutcher, J. D. and Thomas, R. (1964), *Tetrahedron Lett.* 1485–90.

[84] Yamazaki, M., Katoh, F., Ohishi, J. and Koyama, Y. (1972), *Tetrahedron Lett.* 2701–4.

[85] Westley, J. W., Pruess, D. L. and Pitcher, R. G. (1972), *J. Chem. Soc. Chem. Comm.*, 161–2.

[86] Tanabe, M., Hamasaki, T., Suzuki, Y. and Johnson, L. F. (1973), *J. Chem. Soc. Chem. Comm.*, 212–3.

4. Terpenes and steroids

4.1 Introduction

The polyketides form a group of metabolites which are based on patterns of repeating acetate units (Chapter 3). There is another group of metabolites, widespread in nature and rich in diverse chemistry, which is based on another repeating unit: isoprene (*4.1*). Over a

(*4.1*) Isoprene

hundred years ago (*4.1*) began to be identified as a product of thermal decomposition of rubber and other, fragrant natural compounds of low molecular weight. The idea grew that these compounds and many others, generically the terpenes, were formed by head-to-tail linkage of isoprene units. The ideas became encapsulated in what is called the isoprene rule. This relationship of terpene to isoprene can be seen in geraniol (*4.2*), α-terpineol (*4.3*) and γ-cadinene (*4.4*) (dot-

(*4.2*) Geraniol   (*4.3*) α-Terpineol   (*4.4*) γ-Cadinene

ted lines). Exceptions began to appear, however, e.g. artemesia ketone (*4.5*), and notably lanosterol (*4.6*). The assignment of structure (*4.6*) to lanosterol had two fundamental consequences. One was to suggest clearly the course of cholesterol (and steroid) biosynthesis: see below. The second consequence was initiation of a re-examination of the isoprene rule and its reformulation in biogenetic terms, [6] i.e. terpenes are compounds formed as follows: (i) linear combination of isoprene units occurs to give geraniol (*4.2*) (C_{10}), farnesol (*4.9*) (C_{15}), geranylgeraniol (*4.7*) (C_{20}), squalene (*4.8*) (C_{30})*

---

*Squalene is formed by head-on junction of two farnesol units and so obviously the head-to-tail pattern is interrupted (see Section 4.4).

(4.5) Artemesia ketone

(4.6) Lanosterol

(4.7) Geranylgeraniol

(4.8) Squalene

and similar compounds; (ii) other terpenes are derived from these compounds by mechanistically reasonable cyclization and, in some cases, rearrangement reactions. The derivation of α-terpineol (4.3) by cyclization of the geraniol (4.2) skeleton is mechanistically reasonable. The formation of eremorphilone (4.10) can be rationalized as shown in Scheme 4.1, and involves a 1,2-methyl shift (for further examples of such shifts see Section 4.2 and following sections).

(4.9) Farnesol

Ring closure; methyl migration

Scheme 4.1   (4.10) Eremorphilone

The multiples of isoprene units in a terpene serve to classify it: C_{10}, monoterpenes; C_{15}, sesquiterpenes; C_{20}, diterpenes; C_{30}, triterpenes to which the steroids are closely related; C_{25}, sesterpenes. It is a curious thing to note that the isoprene rule, sound and powerfully useful not least for structure elucidation, has *un*natural foundations. Isoprene (4.1) is not a naturally occurring compound. Instead the clay from which the terpenes are so orderly fashioned is isopentenyl pyrophosphate (4.14) and dimethylallyl pyrophosphate (4.15). The latter is seen in many natural compounds, e.g. (4.11), as a 'prenyl'

(4.11)

unit which may also be incorporated as part of a ring system. Mevalonic acid (4.13) is the precursor for isopentenyl pyrophosphate (4.14), and hence other terpenes. The discovery of this was in large measure a serendipitous* one. It was known that (4.13) was a nutrient for bacterial growth and (4.13) was then tried as a steroid precursor with positive results [7]. Detailed later work showed that mevalonic acid is in turn derived, as the (3R)-isomer (4.13) by a major pathway from acetyl-coenzyme A (Scheme 4.2; cf. Section

Scheme 4.2

1.1.2, Scheme 1.2) [2, 9, 10]. (A minor pathway is from the α-amino acid, leucine.) The initial steps involve reactive thio-esters (Co-A esters) and lead to β-hydroxy-β-methylglutaryl-CoA [(4.12) HMG-CoA]. The conversion of (4.12) into mevalonic acid (4.13) is irreversible; the mevalonic acid has no metabolic future except in the formation of terpenes and steroids.

Because of the biological importance of steroids, the main thrust in the investigation of terpene and steroid biosynthesis has been concerned with the latter. These investigations, surely amongst the most notable of biosynthetic studies, are marked by far-seeing intuition, intellectual and practical brilliance, and outstanding results relating to an intricate pathway (Sections 4.2 and 4.4).

4.2   Steroids [10–13]

It was surmised fifty years ago that cholesterol (4.18) could be formed by cyclization of squalene (4.8), first isolated from a species

---

*Serendipity: defined by Horace Walpole as the knack of making happy discoveries by chance (or intuition?).

of shark (*Squalus*). The side-chain of cholesterol, and other steroids, is isoprenoid in appearance and the labelling by [^{14}C]acetate was consistent with such an origin. The labelling pattern in the rings [▲ = labelling sites in (*4.18*) from [1-^{14}C]-labelled material] in conjunction with a consideration of possibilities raised by the structure of lanosterol (*4.6*) suggested that squalene (*4.8*) was folded as shown (in a manner different to the original guess) to give lanosterol (*4.6*) after a series of 1,2-shifts (see Scheme 4.3). Modification of (*4.6*) by

Scheme 4.3

loss essentially of three carbon atoms would give cholesterol (*4.18*). This was supported by showing that squalene was formed *in vivo* from acetate and converted into cholesterol [14, 15]. Importantly, mevalonic acid (*4.13*) was also shown to be a cholesterol precursor with labelling by six units in the appropriate manner. [The most recent results have been obtained with ^{13}C-labelled materials; ● = labelling sites in (*4.18*) from [5-^{13}C]-labelled material. For [2-^{14}C]-labelling see Scheme 4.4. The reader should trace the acetate and mevalonate labels through Schemes 4.2, 4.3 and 4.4 [16].]

Cell-free extracts of liver and yeast were obtained which would synthesize squalene (*4.8*) from mevalonic acid (*4.13*) in the presence of Mg^{2+}, ATP, and NADPH as co-factors. In the absence of NADPH, farnesyl pyrophosphate (*4.19*) accumulated; it was transformed into squalene in the presence of NADPH. In the presence of iodoacetamide as an inhibitor a new and important intermediate, isopentenyl pyrophosphate (*4.14*), was detected [17, 18]. Thus (*4.14*) and (*4.19*) are defined as key staging posts along the route to squalene (*4.8*) and cholesterol (*4.18*).

The cyclization of squalene is aerobic and label from $^{18}O_2$ was incorporated into the C-3 hydroxy-group of cholesterol (*4.18*). The intermediate on which cyclization occurs was identified as squalene-

Mevalonic acid labelling
▲ : 3' – ^{13}C
■ : 4 – ^{13}C

(4.19) Farnesyl pyrophosphate

(4.20)

2,3-oxide [(4.16), absolute stereochemistry as shown] [19–21]. The reasonable sequence of cyclization and migration proposed is shown in Scheme 4.3 (the squalene conformation for cyclization required by the lanosterol stereochemistry is chair-boat-chair and initially a chair for ring D). Its correctness rests on several pieces of key information. Conversion of the mevalonic acid (4.13) into squalene (4.8), involves retention of the (4-pro-R)-hydrogen atom [and loss of the (4-pro-S)-proton; for a discussion of prochirality see Section 1.2.1]. Thus, in the course of biosynthesis by rat liver enzymes, [2-^{14}C, (4R)-^{3}H]-mevalonate [as (4.13)] gave squalene (4.8) with six tritium atoms (^{14}C:^{3}H, 6:6). The derived lanosterol showed a ratio of 6:5; in the mechanism shown (Scheme 4.4, cf. Scheme 4.3) the mevalonoid (4-pro-R)-protons are shown as tritium atoms; one [at C-9 in (4.17)] is

Squalene ^{14}C/T : 6/6
● : label from [2-^{14}C] mevalonate

Cholesterol ^{14}C/T : 5/3

Lanosterol ^{14}C/T : 6/5

Scheme 4.4

lost on formation of lanosterol. The cholesterol formed showed a ratio of 5:3 (one ^{14}C label is inevitably lost as are two tritiums associated with rings A and B). A single tritium atom was located in the nucleus, at C-17α, and two in the side-chain in accord with prediction (Schemes 4.3 and 4.4) [10]. Further evidence is that lanosterol (4.6) obtained from [11, 14-^{3}H$_2$]squalene-2,3-oxide [as (4.16)] in yeast retained essentially all the residual tritium at C-17 in accord with the theory [C-11 tritium becomes the hydrogen atom at C-9 in (*4.17*) and is thus, by the proposed mechanism, lost] [22].

The mechanism shown (Scheme 4.3) involves *two* 1,2-methyl migrations [see (*4.17*)] (from C-8 to C-14, and C-14 to C-13). [3', 4-$^{13}C_2$]Mevalonic acid [as (*4.13*); labels in the *same* molecule] gave cholesterol (*4.20*) from which *di*labelled acetic acid (corresponding to C-13 and attached methyl group) was obtained. This is consistent only with two 1,2-migrations because the methyl group at C-13 must derive from the same molecule of mevalonic acid as C-13 does (i.e. arise from C-14 in (*4.17*)); a 1,3-shift from C-8 to C-13 would have involved a methyl group from a different molecule of mevalonic acid terminating on C-13 [see dotted lines in (*4.20*)], and because of dilution of label within the system, adjacent mevalonate units were unlikely to be labelled. So a 1,3-migration would have given largely singly labelled acetic acid [23, 24].

The C-14 to C-13 methyl migration has been shown to occur with retention of configuration. (This might be expected by analogy with similar stereochemistry in Wagner–Meerwein rearrangements.) This was shown using mevalonic acid chirally labelled with ^3H, ^2H, and ^1H at C-3'; acetic acid from C-13 and C-18 of cholesterol (*4.18*) was isolated and subjected to the usual enzyme analysis: the acetic acid obtained was of the same configuration as the mevalonate (for a detailed discussion of chiral acetic acid see Section 1.2.2) [25].

The bioconversion of lanosterol (*4.6*) into cholesterol (*4.18*) involves most obviously loss of three methyl groups, but also saturation of the side-chain double bond and migration of the $\Delta^{8,9}$ double bond to the $\Delta^{5,6}$ position. The C-4 methyl groups are lost as carbon dioxide [26, 27], the C-14 one as formic acid [28]. It appears that loss occurs first of the methyl group at C-14. This is associated with loss of a 15α proton (Scheme 4.5); subsequent saturation of the new double

Scheme 4.5

bond occurs in a *trans* manner (addition of 14α and 15β protons) [28–30]. Stepwise oxidation of the C-4 methyl groups and loss via a C-3 ketone (loss of C-3 proton: see Scheme 4.4) has been established by detailed investigation (Scheme 4.6), and occurs with the nuclear double bond at either C-7 or C-8 [26, 27].

Scheme 4.6

† Double-bond saturation in the side-chain occurs stereospecifically in the *cis* sense to the *re* face of the double bond: a proton is added to C-24 and a hydride ion from NADPH to C-25. Nuclear double-bond migration is: $\Delta^8 \rightarrow \Delta^7 \rightarrow \Delta^{5,7} \rightarrow \Delta^5$ and involves formation of 7-dehydrocholesterol (*4.23*) as an intermediate with removal of the 5α, C-6α and C-7β protons (information ingeniously gained using chirally tritiated mevalonate). [In ergosterol (*4.21*) biosynthesis the

(4.21) Ergosterol

(4.22) Oestrone

C-7α proton is lost.] Reduction of the 5,7-diene occurs in a *trans* sense but as for side-chain hydrogenation a proton and an NADPH hydrogen is added (C-8β and C-7α, respectively) [31, 32].

† From cholesterol (*4.18*) biosynthesis leads through truncation of the side-chain and other modifications to mammalian steroid hormones, e.g. oestrone (*4.22*) [11, 33]. Vitamin D$_3$ (*4.24*) is obtainable by photochemically mediated electrocyclic ring-opening of 7-dehydrocholesterol (*4.23*), followed by a thermal 1,7-sigmatropic hydrogen shift (Scheme 4.7) [34, 35]. The ecdysone insect moulting

(4.23) 7-Dehydrocholesterol

Scheme 4.7

(4.24) Vitamin D$_3$

hormones, e.g. ecdysterone (*4.25*), are further metabolites of cholesterol which is taken in the insect's diet [36]. Ergosterol (*4.21*)
derives in yeast and fungi from lanosterol (*4.6*) [37].

(*4.25*) Ecdysterone   (*4.26*) = (*4.17*)   (*4.27*) Cycloartenol

The biosynthesis of steroids in photosynthetic organisms proceeds
via cycloartenol (*4.27*) rather than lanosterol (*4.6*). Formation of cycloartenol (*4.27*) can be seen as an alternative way of quenching the
formal carbonium ion (*4.17*) (or enzyme-stabilized equivalent) [see
(*4.26*)]. Tritium n.m.r. analysis of cycloartenol (*4.27*) formed from
squalene-2,3-oxide (*4.16*) with a chiral methyl group at C-6 (^{1}H, ^{2}H,
and a high enrichment of ^{3}H) shows elegantly that cyclopropane
ring-formation occurs with retention of configuration at this carbon
atom [38].

† Plant sterols are characterized by alkyl substituted side-chains.
These substituents and the C-24 methyl group of ergosterol (*4.21*)
have been shown to arise from *S*-adenosylmethionine and by tracing
the fates of individual hydrogen atoms the mechanistic rationale
shown in Scheme 4.8 can be advanced; the slime mould sterol (*4.28*)

Scheme 4.8

retains five methionine protons within its ethyl group, implying formation via route b, whereas poriferasterol (*4.29*) in the alga *Poterio-
ochromonas malhamensis* retains four, thus being formed via route a [39,
40]. For plant sterols side-chain alkylation is an early step in cycloartenol modification whereas for ergosterol (*4.21*) [37] in yeast it
seems to be at a late stage of biosynthesis.

(4.28)

(4.29) Poriferasterol

Ergosterol (*4.21*) and some plant sterols, e.g. (*4.29*), contain a C-22 double bond. Generally the timing of its introduction in relation to other biosynthetic steps is unclear. Moreover, although dehydrogenation is stereospecific, which protons are removed vary with the organism type [39–41].

† One line of plant steroid biosynthesis leads through cholesterol (*4.18*) and pregnenolone (*4.30*) to the cardenolides, e.g. digitoxigenin (*4.31*), with inclusion of an acetate unit [42]. On the other hand, spirostanols, e.g. tigogenin (*4.32*), derive from the intact cholesterol skeleton [43, 44] and the steroidal alkaloids are close relatives [45].

(4.30) Pregnenolone

(4.31) Digitoxigenin

(4.32) Tigogenin

4.3   Pentacyclic triterpenes

A number of groups of triterpenes can be distinguished [6] arising from different ways of discharging an intermediate carbonium ion formalized as (*4.33*) [which is generated by cyclization of squalene-2,3-oxide (*4.16*) in the conformation of a chair (ring A)-chair (B)-chair(C)-boat (initially ring D) (cf. lanosterol formation above)]. This is illustrated for the formation of lupeol (*4.34*) and β-amyrin (*4.35*) in Scheme 4.9. The mechanism shown has been confirmed in the usual, powerful way with tritiated mevalonate samples, in this case $(4R)$-[4-^{3}H]mevalonic acid. This label would appear at the sites shown in (*4.33*) and, in accord with the route shown, appears as illustrated in β-amyrin (*4.35*). Supporting evidence was obtained using [4-^{13}C]mevalonate [46, 47].

Scheme 4.9   (4.35) β-Amyrin

β-Amyrin has been shown to derive from squalene-2,3-oxide [48], but for fernene (*4.36*) which lacks a C-3 hydroxy-group and the protozoan metabolite, tetrahymanol (*4.37*), biosynthesis proceeds through direct protonation of squalene (*4.8*) (tetrahymanol is thus best thought of as having its hydroxy-group at C-21 rather than C-3) [49–51]. The structure of onocerin (*4.39*) suggests that it is formed by cyclization from both ends of squalene-diepoxide (*4.38*).

(4.36) Fernene   (4.37) Tetrahymanol

(4.38)   (4.39) Onocerin

Interestingly it has been shown that the geminal methyl groups at either end of squalene may retain their identity: in soyasapogenol (*4.40*) the C-4 methyl group, but not the hydroxymethyl group, derives from C-2 of mevalonate and in lupeol (*4.34*) the C-22 methyl substituent again arises from C-2 of mevalonate [52, 53].

(4.40) Soyasapogenol

(4.41) Geranyl pyrophosphate

4.4   Squalene [10]

The preceding discussion has indicated the sequence of squalene *(4.8)* biosynthesis as mevalonate *(4.13)* → isopentyl pyrophosphate *(4.14)* ⇆ dimethylallyl pyrophosphate *(4.15)* → geranyl pyrophosphate *(4.41)* → farnesyl pyrophosphate *(4.19)* → squalene *(4.8)*. Each stage involves stereochemical change at one or two carbon atoms. The presence of several prochiral centres in the molecules of this sequence meant that for stereochemical changes to be monitored they had to be chirally labelled with deuterium or tritium: e.g. the condensation of isopentenyl pyrophosphate *(4.14)* with dimethylallyl pyrophosphate *(4.15)* (see Scheme 4.10) involves loss of one of the

Dimethylallyl pyrophosphate, R=H
Geranyl pyrophosphate, R = CH₂

Farnesyl pyrophosphate, R = CH₂

Scheme 4.10

(mevalonoid) C-4 protons. Conversion of labelled mevalonate samples into farnesyl pyrophosphate *(4.19)* and analysis of the *(4.19)*, established that the mevalonoid (4-*pro-S*)-proton [see *(4.13)*] was removed stereospecifically during isomerization of *(4.14)* to *(4.15)* and during successive additions of isopentenyl pyrophosphate *(4.14)* to dimethylallyl pyrophosphate *(4.15)* and *(4.41)* yielding farnesyl pyrophosphate *(4.19)*. Extensive, and quite brilliant, investigation [10] has allowed deduction of the stereochemistry, and hence mechanism, at each stage in the biosynthetic sequence to squalene. (For a detailed discussion the reader is referred to [10].) The pathway to farnesyl pyrophosphate is illustrated in Scheme 4.10; it is to be noted that reaction between *(4.14)* and *(4.15)* results in normal inversion of configuration at C-5 (mevalonate numbering) of the latter and in all successive steps. Addition to the double bond of isopentenyl pyrophosphate is to the same side as proton removal. Chemical experience suggests that this would be more favourable if the opposite were true and so a two-step mechanism, involving some enzyme-linked X-H group, has been proposed (Scheme 4.10). Most recently using pig liver enzymes the question of the stereochemistry involved at C-4 in the interconversion of dimethylallyl pyrophosphate and isopentenyl pyrophosphate has been examined. $(2R)$-[2-^{3}H]Mevalonate (4.42) gave isopentenyl pyrophosphate (4.43). This, in a deuterium oxide medium, would give dimethylallyl pyrophosphate (4.44) with chiral methyl group having the shown, or opposite, stereochemistry. Analysis of this methyl group as chiral acetic acid [as (4.46)] (see Section 1.2.2) derived from farnesyl pyrophosphate

(4.42) (4.43) (4.44)

(4.46) (4.45)

(4.45) demonstrated that the dimethylallyl pyrophosphate had the stereochemistry shown in (4.44). Thus addition of the deuteron is to the re-face of (4.43) and is of opposite stereochemistry to that observed in the association of C_5 units in farnesyl pyrophosphate formation. Earlier results, alluded to above, establish that the same C-4 proton is lost in isomerization and condensation (Scheme 4.10). In the isomerization a simple one-step mechanism involving $trans$ removal and addition of protons is now possible [54].

In the formation of squalene $[(4.8) = (4.47)]$ units of farnesyl pyrophosphate come together not head-to-tail as in their formation, but 'head-on'. In this process the (1-pro-S)-proton in one of the farnesyl pyrophosphate units (A) (Scheme 4.11) is lost to be replaced

(A)   (B)   NADPH (4.47) Squalene

Scheme 4.11

with retention of configuration by a hydrogen from NADPH [the (4-pro-S)-proton] [10, 11, 55, 56]. It is interesting to note that squalene, a symmetrical molecule, is thus formed in an unsymmetrical way.

The next step in understanding squalene biosynthesis depended on the isolation, from yeast and from rat liver microsomal incubations in the absence of NADPH, of a cyclopropyl compound, presqualene pyrophosphate (*4.48*); it is established as an intermediate in squalene biosynthesis (in micromosal preparations it is converted into squalene in the presence of NADPH) [57–60]. A reasonable mechanism for the biosynthesis of squalene (*4.47*) via presqualene pyrophosphate (*4.48*) is shown in Scheme 4.12 [60–63].

Scheme 4.12

4.5 Monoterpenes [64]

The relationship of cyclic monoterpenes, e.g. (*4.3*) and (*4.53*), to geranyl pyrophosphate (*4.41*) is an obvious one. The *trans* double bond in (*4.41*) means that (*4.41*) cannot cyclize directly to give monoterpenes such as (*4.53*), and neryl pyrophosphate (*4.51*) may be more directly involved in biosynthesis. [A cell-free preparation of *Mentha piperita* has been obtained which will catalyse the conversion of neryl pyrophosphate (*4.51*) into α-terpineol (*4.3*) [65].] The conversion of geraniol (*4.2*) into nerol (*4.49*) is well known and involves a stereospecific proton removal from C-1; loss of a proton indicates that the aldehyde (*4.50*) is involved in double-bond isomerization [66]. Initiation of cyclic monoterpene formation can be seen as

(*4.49*) R = CH₂OH
(*4.50*) R = CHO

(*4.51*) Neryl pyrophosphate

(*4.52*)

(*4.53*)

(*4.54*)

occurring through the carbonium ion (4.52) [6]. An interesting observation is that (+)-car-3-ene derives as shown in (4.53), which is the reverse of what was originally thought, i.e. (4.54) [● = [2-¹⁴C]mevalonate label in (4.52) and (4.53)] [67].

Monoterpenes with a rearranged skeleton are interesting. Artemesia ketone (4.55) is one such compound. It has been shown to derive from [2-¹⁴C]mevalonate consistent with biosynthesis from a compound of the chrysanthemyl type [as (4.56)] which is an analogue of presqualene alcohol [as (4.48)]. Artemesia ketone was also labelled by isopentenyl pyrophosphate (4.14) but not geraniol (4.2) [68]. [As commonly observed with monoterpenes, mevalonate gave unequal labelling of the two C_5 units. This may be explained generally in terms of pools of (4.14) and (4.15) being of different sizes and accessibility. A further general problem is that of obtaining significant incorporation of mevalonate.] Chrysanthemic acid (4.57) derives from chrysanthemyl alcohol (4.56) but the mechanism of ring closure and the nature of earlier intermediates is unknown [69].

(4.55) Artemesia ketone   (4.56) Chrysanthemyl alcohol   (4.57) Chrysanthemic acid

(4.58) Plumieride   (4.59) Loganin

† In this area of sparse experimental results it is interesting to note genetic studies on the biosynthesis of some terpenes [70].

† Iridoids, e.g. plumieride (4.58) [71] and loganin (4.59), have been the subject of extensive and fruitful study. In particular this is true for the iridoid fragment that is found in terpenoid indole alkaloids. For a discussion the reader is referred to Section 6.6.2.

4.6 Sesquiterpenes [72]

The enzyme, farnesyl pyrophosphate synthetase (prenyl transferase), is responsible for the condensation of (4.14) with (4.15) to give geranyl pyrophosphate (4.41). The same enzyme mediates addition of a further molecule of (4.14) to (4.41) yielding 2-*trans*-farnesyl pyrophosphate (4.19). This is the basic unit for the elaboration of the structurally diverse sesquiterpenes. The results obtained on biosynthesis are as interesting as the sesquiterpene structures. The 2-*cis* isomer (*4.65*) of (*4.19*), required for forming some sesquiterpenes (see Scheme 4.13) may apparently be formed by isomerization of (*4.63*) [66, 73].

Formation of abscisic acid (*4.62*), a plant growth regulator, is established to be from mevalonic acid (*4.13*) and involves loss of the (4-*pro-S*)-proton and (two-thirds) retention of the (4-*pro-R*)-proton (at C-2). This is consistent with formation of (*4.62*), with its terminal

(*4.60*) Farnesol   (*4.61*)   (*4.62*) Abscisic acid

cis double bond, from *trans*-farnesol (*4.60*) with subsequent isomerization [terpenoid *trans* and *cis* double bonds involve loss of the mevalonoid (4-*pro-S*)-proton; the *cis* double bonds in rubber are formed with loss of the (4-*pro-R*)-proton]. Mevalonic acid samples chirally labelled with tritium at C-2 and C-5 gave results which indicate that the C-4,5 double bond introduced during biotransformation of [(*4.60*) = (*4.63*)] into abscisic acid (*4.62*) occurs with *trans* removal of hydrogen. Similar results have been observed in carotenoid biosynthesis.

It is *a priori* possible that (*4.62*) is a carotenoid [cf. the structure (*4.124*) for β-carotene] degradation product but it has been shown that phytoene (*4.122*) is not a precursor for (*4.62*) (in avocado fruit) although it is as usual incorporated into carotenoids (Section 4.9). The observation that the abscisic acid concentration increases twenty-five fold in wilting wheat, has been cleverly exploited in examining the epoxide (*4.61*) as a precursor (fed as a mixture with the isomeric epoxide). A nine-times improvement in incorporation was observed and it was shown that the C-1' oxygen atom was derived from the epoxide oxygen in (*4.61*). Further results confirmed that (*4.61*), with stereochemistry shown, is the precursor for abscisic acid (*4.62*). Finally, it is to be noted that formation of abscisic acid (*4.62*) and a related metabolite, phaseic acid, involves distinction being kept between C-3' and C-2 of mevalonate in the C-6' methyl groups [74].

Germacrene C (*4.64*) has been shown to derive from mevalonate and 2-*trans*-farnesol (*4.60*). Its formation can be seen to be the result of displacement of pyrophosphate from C-1 of farnesyl pyrophosphate (*4.63*) by the distal double bond, Scheme 4.13. An oxygenated relative of (*4.64*), ageratriol has been shown to derive similarly via oxygenated intermediates [75, 76]. Further cyclization of the germacrene skeleton [as (*4.64*)] would afford compounds of type (*4.4*). On the other hand caryophyllene (*4.66*), known to be derived from mevalonate, is expected to derive from 2-*cis*-farnesol (*4.65*) in a dif-

(4.63) 2-trans-Farnesyl
pyrophosphate

(4.64) Germacrene

(4.65) 2-cis Farnesyl
pyrophosphate

(4.66) Caryophyllene

Scheme 4.13

(4.67) Carotol

ferent manner (Scheme 4.13) [77]. Carotol (4.67) is also expected to derive from 2-cis-farnesol, see Scheme 4.13; the acetate labelling pattern is consistent with the path shown [78].

Petasin (4.68) although similar to γ-cadinene (4.4) differs from it in the siting of one methyl group. A plausible mechanism for its formation, involves a methyl shift from C-10 to C-5 as shown (Scheme 4.14, cf. Scheme 4.1). Normal labelling of the skeleton of (4.68) with [2-^{14}C]mevalonate was observed (isopropyl group, C-3, and C-9).

Scheme 4.14

(4.68) Petasin

Tritium from (4-R)[4-^{3}H]mevalonate in particular appeared at C-4 indicating clearly that methyl migration is attended by a 1,2-proton shift. The proposed methyl migration is supported by results with [1,2-^{13}C$_2$]acetate in the biosynthesis of capsidiol (4.69) [no coupling between C-5 and C-15, therefore they are from separate mevalonate units, see (4.69)] [79]. A further point of interest with regard to petasin biosynthesis, studied in *Petasites hybridus*, was the use of an enzyme inhibitor which suppressed the biosynthesis of phytosterols and improved the mevalonate incorporation into (4.68). (A significant enhancement of mevalonate incorporation into caryophyllene in cut stems of the peppermint plant was observed with added sucrose.)

† 2-cis-Farnesol [as (4.65)] is a precursor for γ-bisabolene (4.70) in tissue cultures. A related compound paniculide B has been shown by [1,2-^{13}C$_2$]acetate labelling to be formed with similar folding of the

(4.69) Capsidiol

(4.70) γ-Bisabolene

cf. Scheme 4.14

(4.71) Lubimin

farnesyl chain [80]. [^{13}C]Acetate labelling indicates that lubimin (4.71) is formed as shown [81].

† The skeleton of fumagillin (4.73), obtained from *Aspergillus fumigatus*, is not classically isoprenoid, but the deduced acetate and mevalonate labelling patterns indicate it to be a sesquiterpene. Its formation from farnesol has been rationalized as shown in Scheme 4.15, with (4.72), cf. (4.70), as a key intermediate. Powerful supplementary information has been obtained for the related metabolite, ovalicin (4.74) with [3,4-^{13}C$_2$]mevalonate [labelling of C-1 + C-6, C-10 + C-11, by respectively, C-4 and C-3 of single molecules of labelled mevalonate; C-7 (and C-3) were deduced to be part of a fragmented mevalonate unit: see ● positions in Scheme 4.15] and [1,2-^{13}C$_2$]acetate (showed incorporation of six intact acetate units and therefore no methyl migrations had occurred). The data are consistent with the pathway shown in Scheme 4.15 [82].

(4.72)

(4.74) Ovalicin

Scheme 4.15

(4.73) Fumagillin

† The C$_7$ side-chain of the *Penicillium* metabolite, mycophenolic acid (4.77), has been shown to derive from mevalonate. The obviously polyketide nucleus has its origins in acetate, and the remaining carbons from methionine [marked ■ in (4.77)]. The phthalide (4.75) is a precursor. After adding it to the culture medium a new, farnesyl based, metabolite (4.76), was isolated which was converted efficiently into (4.77) by the organism. The biosynthetic pathway follows as that shown [83, 84].

(4.75)   (4.76)   (4.77) Mycophenolic acid

Coriamyrtin (4.78), tutin (4.79), picrotoxinin (4.80) (part of the complex metabolite, picrotoxin) and the alkaloid, dendrobine (4.81), are interesting sesquiterpenes which all embrace the structure (4.86). Labelling patterns in (4.78) and (4.79) from [2-^{14}C]- and [4-^{14}C]-mevalonate and the specific incorporation of labelled copaborneol (4.82; ⋏⋏⋏: bond broken) indicates the pathway to these compounds

(4.78) R=H, Coriamyrtin
(4.79) R=OH, Tutin   (4.80) Picrotoxinin   (4.81) Dendrobine   (4.82)

shown in Scheme 4.16. Additional information is available on dendrobine (4.81) biosynthesis and here it was shown that biosynthesis was accompanied by a 1,3-hydrogen shift, see (4.84) [H$_R$:a

(4.83)   (4.84)   (4.85)   (4.86)

Scheme 4.16

5-^{3}H$_2$ mevalonate label located at C-8 in (4.81); five out of the six labels were retained]. A 1,2-shift of hydrogen was excluded in tutin biosynthesis, 2-*trans*- rather than 2-*cis*-farnesol is a precursor for dendrobine (4.81) and further results show that it is the farnesol (1-*pro-R*)-hydrogen atom which migrates to C-8 in (4.81). The deduced pathway to dendrobine and related sesquiterpenes is summarized in Scheme 4.16 (cf. Scheme 4.17) [85–88].

(4.87) ≡ (4.85)   (4.88) cf (4.82)   (4.89) Sativene

Scheme 4.17

† In the biosynthesis of sativene (*4.89*) all six of the C-5 mevalonate protons are retained and one of these, a (5-*pro-R*)-proton as in dendrobine formation, migrates to quench the carbonium ion on the isopropyl group in (*4.84*). The data are consistent with a pathway as shown in Scheme 4.17 which parallels that in Scheme 4.16. Interestingly, the isopropyl methyl groups retain their identity from mevalonate unlike tutin (*4.79*) which in this resembles iridoid terpenes. Loss or retention of identity in the methyl groups here may be interpreted as being the result of whether or not rotation of the isopropyl group occurs in (*4.84*) before quenching of the planar carbonium ion [66].

† (+)-Longifolene (*4.90*) can be seen to arise from (*4.83*), this time through an intermediate 11-membered, rather than a 10-membered [as (*4.84*)], ring. A 1,3-hydrogen shift is again observed and it is the

Farnesol

Scheme 4.18

(*4.90*) (+) – Longifolene

● = label from [2-^{14}C]mevalonate

(5-*pro-R*)-hydrogen which again migrates (Scheme 4.18). The formation of the fungal metabolite, avocettin (*4.92*), may *a priori* be thought of as being via (*4.84*) like other sesquiterpenes discussed above (Schemes 4.16 and 4.17). However, it is the mevalonoid (5-*pro-S*)-proton which migrates in this case. This is an important difference and the formation of avocettin (*4.92*), sativene (*4.89*), coriamyrtin (*4.78*) through dendrobine (*4.81*), and longifolene (*4.90*) has been very carefully correlated with the conformation adopted by (*4.83*), which has specifically either the 2-*cis* or 2-*trans* configuration, during cyclization [as (*4.93*)]. One result is the particular hydrogen shifts observed. The other is the eventual stereochemistry of

(*4.91*)

(*4.92*) Avocettin

(*4.93*)

(*4.94*) Culmorin

the sesquiterpene formed. (For a detailed discussion the reader is referred to [66].) In the biosynthesis of (−)-longifolene it is the mevalonoid (5-*pro-S*)-hydrogen which migrates [66, 89]. A similar migration is observed in culmorin (*4.94*) biosynthesis [90].

† [1,2-^{13}C$_2$]Acetate gave a labelling pattern in 5-dihydrocoriolin C (*4.96*) which could be clearly interpreted in terms of a pathway based on the humulene skeleton (*4.95*) (Scheme 4.19). A similar route to related compounds, hirsutic and complicatic acids, and the illudins, is likely [91–94].

(4.95) → Scheme 4.19 → (4.96)

† At first sight trichothecin (4.98) and helicobasidin [(5.45); p. 86] (for further discussion of helicobasidin biosynthesis, see Section 5.2) do not seem to be related, but, it turns out, they are both based on the skeleton (4.97). Studies on the incorporation, particularly of specifically tritiated mevalonate samples into (4.98) and related compounds, establish a complex sequence of proton and methyl shifts during the course of biosynthesis. Further information has been obtained by examining new tricothecin-like metabolites as precursors for (4.98) and biosynthesis proceeds as shown briefly in Scheme 4.20 [95].

(4.97)

Scheme 4.20   (4.98) Trichothecin

† Gossypol (4.99) is clearly formed by phenol oxidative coupling (Section 1.3.1) of two molecules of (4.100). Gosspyol was shown to derive from mevalonate. Material derived from three radioactive precursors was in turn degraded to gossic acid (4.101) to distinguish the various ways in which a farnesol chain could fold to give (4.100). [2-^{14}C]Mevalonate gave (4.101) with the same radioactivity as (4.99), therefore [(4.102); ● = mevalonate label] is excluded. [2-^{14}C]-Geraniol and -nerol gave radioactive (4.101) but [2-^{14}C]farnesol did not, thus excluding (4.103) and indicating (4.104) as the manner of folding (▲ = geraniol, ■ = farnesol and ● = mevalonate label). Moreover,

(4.99) Gossypol   (4.100)   (4.101)

(4.102)   (4.103)   (4.104)

as required by the manner of folding, the favoured precursor is
2-*cis*-6-*cis*-farnesol (*4.104*) [96].

4.7 Diterpenes

The diterpenes are elaborations of geranylgeranyl pyrophosphate
(*4.105*). Cyclization may occur to give diterpenes, in a manner similar to that for sesquiterpenes discussed above, by attack of the distal
double bond as shown in (*4.105*). An example is found in the biosynthesis of fusicoccin (*4.106*). The labelling pattern of (*4.106*), derived
from [3-^{13}C]- and (4R)-[4-^{3}H]-mevalonic acid, is consistent with the
route shown in Scheme 4.21. Mevalonic acid labelled with ^{13}C and

(*4.105*) Geranylgeranyl
pyrophosphate

Scheme 4.21

(*4 106*) Fusicoccin

^{2}H has been used ingeniously to confirm the 1,2-shifts of protons in
fusicoccin biosynthesis (by ^{13}C n.m.r. analysis) [97, 98].

An alternative path to diterpenes has some similarity to that
which gives the triterpenes and steroids, as (*4.105*) to (*4.107*) in
Scheme 4.22. No epoxide is involved here though, nor is the constant

Geranyl geranyl pyrophosphate
(*4.105*)

(*4.107*)

(*4.110*) Aphidicolin

(*4.108*) R = OH } Virescenols
(*4.109*) R = H }

Scheme 4.22

absolute stereochemistry of the triterpenoid–steroid group maintained in the diterpenes.

Simple derivatives of (4.107), formed following a second cyclization, are virescenols A (4.108) and B (4.109) and aphidicolin (4.110).
Use, in particular, of [1,2-^{13}C$_2$]acetate as precursor has established
the biosynthetic pathway shown in Scheme 4.22 [99, 100].

† Detailed study has been carried out on the biosynthesis of the
fungal metabolite, rosenonolactone (4.111). [^{14}C]Acetate and
[^{14}C]mevalonate labelling is consistent with the path shown in
Scheme 4.23, in which a methyl group migrates from C-10 to C-9.

(= 4.107)　　　　　Scheme 4.23　　　　(4.111) Rosenonolactone

There is also a proposed proton shift from C-9 to C-8. The correctness of this proposal was demonstrated when a mevalonoid (4-*pro*-
R)-tritium atom was found at C-8 (incorporation of other
[^{3}H]mevalonates also excluded $\Delta^{1(10)}$, $\Delta^{5(10)}$, and $\Delta^{5(6)}$ intermediates)
[101]. More extensive migration and also bond fracture within
(4.112) [the carbonium ion preceding (4.107)] is thought to occur in
the biosynthesis of pleuromutilin (4.113). Again it is the mevalonoid
(4-*pro*-*R*)-hydrogen which migrates from C-9 to C-8, and in a subsequent step (see Scheme 4.24) it is a C-5 (*pro*-*S*)-proton which moves
from C-11 to C-4 (the labels from [2-^{14}C]mevalonate = ●) [102].

(4.113) Pleuromutilin

Scheme 4.24

The gibberellins, e.g. gibberellic acid (4.117), first isolated from
the fungus, *Gibberella fujikuroi*, are important plant-growth hormones.
Labelling by [2-^{14}C]mevalonate and [1-^{14}C]acetate established
(4.117) to be a modified diterpene. A number of kauranoid diterpenes, including ent-kaurene (4.114), were found with gibberellic
acid (4.117) in *G. fujikuroi*. This finding provided an important clue
to the course of gibberellic acid (4.117) biosynthesis and (4.114) was

(4.114) Ent-kaurene   (4.115)   (4.116)

(4.117) Gibberellic acid

Scheme 4.25

then confirmed as a precursor for (*4.117*). A soluble enzyme system has also been obtained from fungal and plant sources which will effect the conversion (*4.105*) → (*4.114*). Biosynthesis beyond (*4.114*) involves stepwise oxidation of one of the gem-dimethyl groups, and then hydroxylation at C-7 to give (*4.115*). Ring contraction then occurs with proton loss from C-6.

Gibberellin A_{12} aldehyde (*4.116*) is the first detectable gibbane intermediate in *G. fujikuroi*. From it a web of oxidation reactions leads through to various gibberellins including gibberellic acid (*4.117*), which also involves loss of the C-10 methyl group, probably via a carboxy-function [103–106].

4.8 Sesterpenes [107]
† The ophiobolins are examples of this relatively small class of terpenes. Ophiobolin F (*4.119*) has been shown to derive from geranylfarnesyl pyrophosphate (*4.118*). During biosynthesis a C-2 (*pro-R*)-mevalonoid hydrogen undergoes a stereospecific 1,5-shift from C-8 to C-15 (see Scheme 4.26).

(4.118) Geranylfarnesyl   Scheme 4.26   (4.119) Ophiobolin F
pyrophosphate

4.9 Carotenoids and vitamin A [3, 5, 108]
Most of the natural carotenoid pigments are tetraterpenes, being formed from two C_{20} geranylgeranyl pyrophosphate units through phytoene (*4.122*). The mechanism of phytoene formation has much in common with squalene biosynthesis. In particular, head-on fusion of the two C_{20} units occurs via prephytoene pyrophosphate (*4.120*), analogous to presqualene pyrophosphate (*4.48*) formation from two

2 x Geranylgeranyl pyrophosphate *(4.105)*

(4.120) Prephytoene pyrophosphate

(4.121)

(4.122) Phytoene

(4.123) Lycopene

C_{15} units (Scheme 4.12). Formation and collapse of *(4.48)* and *(4.120)* appear to be similar, the only apparent difference being in the last step: the carbonium ion *(4.121)* is quenched by proton loss to give phytoene *(4.122)*, whereas in squalene formation the corresponding ion is neutralized by hydride donation from NADPH [60].

Most of the phytoene produced *in vivo* appears to be the 15,15'-*cis*-isomer *(4.122)*. Formation of *(4.122)* involves loss of the (1-*pro-S*)-proton from each of the two molecules of *(4.105)*. In some bacteria the 15,15'-*trans* compound is produced by loss of the (1-*pro-S*)-proton from one molecule of *(4.105)* and the (1-*pro-R*)-proton from the other [at the stage of *(4.121)*].

Desaturation of phytoene *(4.122)* occurs in a stepwise manner, each step extending the conjugation of the system, and leading finally to lycopene *(4.123)* (the desaturation sequence is $\Delta^{11,12}$, then $\Delta^{7,8}$ or $\Delta^{11',12'}$, then respectively $\Delta^{11',12'}$ or $\Delta^{7,8}$, then $\Delta^{7',8'}$). The stereochemistry of hydrogen elimination has been shown to be *trans* in experiments with mevalonate *(4.13)* stereospecifically tritiated at C-2 and C-5 [corresponds, respectively, to C-8 and C-7 in *(4.122)*, for example] [109, 110].

Reactions at the C-1,2 double bond of lycopene *(4.123)* leads to a series of acyclic carotenoids characteristic of photosynthetic bacteria, or by cyclization to the mono- and bi-cyclic carotenoids typical of plants. Cyclization is believed to be initiated by protonation at C-2 and to proceed as shown in Scheme 4.27; the three ring types, β, ε

β-ring

γ-ring

ε-ring

Scheme 4.27

and γ, are not interconverted. The biosynthesis of β-carotene *(4.124)* proceeds by two successive reactions to give two β-rings (Scheme 4.27). α-Carotene, on the other hand, is formed by cyclization to give a β-type ring and then one of the ε-type (Scheme 4.27). In certain non-photosynthetic bacteria cyclization may be initiated by an electrophilic species resulting in C_{45} or C_{50} carotenoids, e.g. *(4.126)*.

(4.124) R = H, β-Carotene
(4.125) R = OH, Zeaxanthin

(4.126)

In the cyclization of phytoene *(4.122)* a particular stereochemistry is expected for proton and carbon addition to the C-1 double bond. $[2-^{13}C]$Mevalonate labels the (E)-methyl group at C-1 in lycopene $[(4.127) = (4.123);$ ● = label] and the 1α-methyl group in zeaxanthin $[(4.128) = (4.125)]$ (see Scheme 4.28). Zeaxanthin formed in bacterial cells suspended in deuterium oxide had a 2β-deuteron. It follows that cyclization occurs as shown in Scheme 4.28 [111]. The stereochemistry in the C_{50} carotenoids, e.g. *(4.126)*, implies a different manner of addition to the C-1 double bond.

(4.127)   *(4.128)*

Scheme 4.28

†   Carotenoids found in photosynthetic bacteria may derive by water or hydrogen addition across the C-1 double bond. Since their formation is inhibited by the same substances as inhibit carotenoid cyclization, it may be concluded that these additions and cyclization are similar: hydrogen and water addition initiated by protonation at C-2.

†   Modification of the basic carotenoid skeletons occurs to give a variety of metabolites. The most important reaction is C-3 hydroxylation in cyclic carotenoids [as in *(4.125)*]. In plants and bacteria, it has been shown that zeaxanthin *(4.125)* is formed by hydroxylation of β-carotene *(4.124)*. The reaction is typical of a mixed-function oxidase: the hydroxyl oxygen comes from molecule oxygen and the hydroxylation occurs with retention of stereochemistry (see Section 1.2.3).

β-Carotene
(4.124)

(4.129)

(4.130) R = CHO, Retinaldehyde
(4.131) R = CH₂OH, Vitamin A₁

The most important carotenoid metabolites in animals are the vitamins A: vitamin A₁ (4.131), its 3,4-didehydro-derivative (vitamin A₂), retinaldehyde (4.130) and its 3,4-didehydro-derivative. These vitamins are the basis of rhodopsin and other visual pigments. Retinaldehyde is formed by oxidative cleavage of β-carotene via the peroxide (4.129) and the reaction is catalysed by an enzyme in the intestinal mucosa.

References

Further reading: [1]–[5].

[1] *Natural Substances Formed Biologically from Mevalonic Acid*, (1970), (ed. T. W. Goodwin) Academic Press, New York.
[2] Goodwin, T. W. (1971), in *Rodd's Chemistry of Carbon Compounds*, 2nd Ed. (ed. S. Coffey), vol. IIE, pp. 54–137.
[3] Goodwin, T. W. (1974), in *Rodd's Chemistry of Carbon Compounds*, vol. II Supplement, pp. 237–89.
[4] Hanson, J. R. (1979), in *Comprehensive Organic Chemistry* (ed. D. H. R. Barton and W. D. Ollis), Pergamon, Oxford, vol. 5, pp. 989–1023.
[5] Britton, G. (1979), in *Comprehensive Organic Chemistry* (ed. D. H. R. Barton and W. D. Ollis), Pergamon, Oxford, vol. 5, pp. 1025–42.
[6] Ruzicka, L. (1959), *Proc. Chem. Soc.*, 341–60.
[7] Tavormina, P. A. and Gibbs, M. H. (1956), *J. Amer. Chem. Soc.*, **78**, 6210.
[8] Cornforth, J. W. and Cornforth, R. H. (1970), in *Natural Substances Formed Biologically from Mevalonic Acid* (ed. T. W. Goodwin), Academic Press, New York, pp. 5–15.
[9] Rétey, J., von Stetten, E., Coy, U. and Lynen, F. (1970), *Eur. J. Biochem.*, **15**, 72–6.
[10] Popjak, G. and Cornforth, J. W. (1966), *Biochem. J.*, **101**, 553–68.
[11] Clayton, R. B. (1965), *Quart. Rev. Chem. Soc.*, **19**, 168–230.
[12] Mulheim, L. J. and Ramm, P. J. (1972), *Chem. Soc. Rev.*, **1**, 259–91.
[13] Goad, L. J. (1970), in *Natural Substances Formed Biologically from Mevalonic Acid* (ed. T. W. Goodwin), Academic Press, New York, pp. 45–77.
[14] Woodward, R. B. and Bloch, K. (1953), *J. Amer. Chem. Soc.*, **75**, 2023–4.

[15] Cornforth, J. W., Gore, I. and Popják, G. (1957), *Biochem. J.*, **65**, 94–109.

[16] Popják, G., Edmond, J., Anet, F. A. L. and Easton, N. R. jun., (1977), *J. Amer. Chem. Soc.*, **99**, 931–5.

[17] Schechter, I. and Bloch, K. (1971), *J. Biol. Chem.*, **246**, 7690–6.

[18] *Methods in Enzymology* (1969), (ed. R. B. Clayton), Academic Press, New York, vol. 15.

[19] van Tamelen, E. E., Willet, J. D., Clayton, R. B. and Lord, K. E. (1966), *J. Amer. Chem. Soc.*, **88**, 4752–4.

[20] Corey, E. J., Russey, W. E., Ortiz de Montellano, P. R. (1966), *J. Amer. Chem. Soc.*, **88**, 4750–1.

[21] van Tamelen, E. E. and Hopla, R. E. (1979), *J. Amer. Chem. Soc.*, **101**, 6112–4.

[22] Barton, D. H. R., Mellows, G., Widdowson, D. A. and Wright, J. J. (1971), *J. Chem. Soc. (C)*, 1142–8.

[23] Cornforth, J. W., Cornforth, R. H., Pelter, A., Horning, M. G. and Popják, G. (1959), *Tetrahedron*, **5**, 311–39.

[24] Mandgal, R. K., Tchen, T. T. and Bloch, K. (1958), *J. Amer. Chem. Soc.*, **80**, 2589–90.

[25] Clifford, K. H. and Phillips, G. T. (1976), *Eur. J. Biochem.*, **61**, 271–86.

[26] Miller, W. L. and Gaylor, J. L. (1970), *J. Biol. Chem.*, **245**, 5375–81.

[27] Hornby, G. M. and Boyd, G. S. (1970), *Biochem. Biophys. Res. Comm.*, **40**, 1452–4.

[28] Alexander, K., Akhtar, M., Boar, R. B., McGhie, J. F. and Barton, D. H. R. (1972), *J. Chem. Soc. Chem. Comm.*, 383–5.

[29] Caspi, E., Ramm, P. J. and Gain, R. E. (1969), *J. Amer. Chem. Soc.*, **91**, 4012–3.

[30] Ramm, P. J. and Caspi, E. (1969), *J. Biol. Chem.*, **244**, 6064–73.

[31] Aberhart, D. J. and Caspi, E. (1971), *J. Biol. Chem.*, **246**, 1387–92.

[32] Wilton, D. C. and Akhtar, M. (1970), *Biochem. J.*, **116**, 337–9.

[33] Sih, C. J. and Whitlock, H. W. jun., (1968), *Ann. Rev. Biochem.*, **37**, 661–94.

[34] Georghiu, P. E. (1977), *Chem. Soc. Rev.*, **6**, 83–107.

[35] de Luca, H. F. and Schnoes, H. K. (1976), *Ann. Rev. Biochem.*, **45**, 631–66.

[36] Rees, H. H. and Goodwin, T. W. (1974), *Biochem. Soc. Trans.*, **2**, 1027–32.

[37] Barton, D. H. R., Corrie, J. E. T., Marshall, P. J. and Widdowson, D. A. (1973), *Bio-org. Chem.*, **2**, 363–73.

[38] Altman, L. J., Han, C. Y., Bertolino, A., Handy, G., Laungani, D., Muller, W., Schwatz, S., Shanker, D., de Wolf, W. H. and Yang, F. (1978), *J. Amer. Chem. Soc.*, **100**, 3235–7.

[39] Goad, L. J. and Goodwin, T. W. (1972), *Progr. Phytochem.*, **3**, 113–98.

[40] Knights, B. A. (1973), *Chem. Brit.*, **9**, 106–11.

[41] Bimpson, T., Goad, L. J. and Goodwin, T. W. (1969), *Chem. Comm.*, 297–8.

[42] Caspi, E. and Hornby, G. M. (1968), *Phytochemistry*, **7**, 423–7.

[43] Tschesche, R., Hulpke, H. and Fritz, R. (1968), *Phytochemistry*, **7**, 2021–6.

[44] Tschesche, R. and Spindler, M. (1978), *Phytochemistry*, **17**, 251–5.
[45] Herbert, R. B. (1979), in *The Alkaloids (Specialist Periodical Reports)*, (ed. M. F. Grundon), The Chemical Society, London, vol. 9, pp. 27–8; and earlier volumes in this series.
[46] Seo, S., Tomita, Y. and Tori, K. (1975), *J. Chem. Soc. Chem. Comm.*, 270–1.
[47] Rees, H. H., Britton, G. and Goodwin, T. W. (1968), *Biochem. J.*, **106**, 659–65.
[48] Barton, D. H. R., Jarman, T. R., Watson, K. G., Widdowson, D. A., Boar, R. B. and Damps, K. (1974), *J. Chem. Soc. Chem. Comm.*, 861–2.
[49] Caspi, E., Zander, J. M., Greig, J. B., Mallory, F. B., Conner, R. L. and Landrey, J. B. (1968), *J. Amer. Chem. Soc.*, **90**, 3563–4.
[50] Caspi, E., Greig, J. B. and Zander, J. M. (1968), *J. Biol. Chem.*, **109**, 931–2.
[51] Barton, D. H. R., Gosden, A. F., Mellows, G. and Widdowson, D. A. (1969), *Chem. Comm.*, 185–6.
[52] Arigoni, D. (1958), *Experientia*, **14**, 153–5.
[53] Ruzicka, L. (1963), *Pure Appl. Chem.*, **6**, 493–523.
[54] Clifford, K., Cornforth, J. W., Mallaby, R. and Phillips, G. T. (1971), *J. Chem. Soc. Chem. Comm.*, 1599–600.
[55] Cornforth, J. W. (1969), *Quart. Rev. Chem. Soc.*, **23**, 125–40.
[56] Beytia, E., Qureshi, A. A. and Porter, J. W. (1973), *J. Biol. Chem.*, **248**, 1856–67.
[57] Muscio, F., Carlson, J. P., Kuehl, L. and Rilling, H. C. (1974), *J. Biol. Chem.*, **249**, 3746–9.
[58] Popják, G., Ngan, H.-L. and Agnew, W. (1975), *Bio-org. Chem.*, **4**, 279–89.
[59] Ortiz de Montellano, P. R., Castillo, R., Vinson, W. and Wei, J. S. (1976), *J. Amer. Chem. Soc.*, **98**, 3020–1.
[60] Altman, L. J., Kowerski, R. C. and Laungani, D. P. (1978), *J. Amer. Chem. Soc.*, **100**, 6174–82.
[61] Rilling, H. C., Poulter, C. D., Epstein, W. W. and Larsen, B. (1971), *J. Amer. Chem. Soc.*, **93**, 1783–5.
[62] van Tamelen, E. E. and Schwartz, M. A. (1971), *J. Amer. Chem. Soc.*, pp. 1780–2.
[63] Cornforth, J. W. (1973), *Chem. Soc. Rev.*, **2**, 1–20.
[64] Banthorpe, D. V., Charlwood, B. V. and Francis, M. J. O. (1972), *Chem. Rev.*, **72**, 115–49.
[65] Croteau, R., Burbott, A. J. and Loomis, W. D. (1973), *Biochem. Biophys. Res. Comm.*, **50**, 1006–12.
[66] Arigoni, D. (1975), *Pure Appl. Chem.*, **41**, 219–45.
[67] Banthorpe, D. V. and Ekundayo, O. (1976), *Phytochemistry*, **15**, 109–12.
[68] Banthorpe, D. V., Doonan, S. and Gutowski, J. A. (1977), *Phytochemistry*, **16**, 85–92.
[69] Pattenden, G., Popplestone, C. R. and Storer, R. (1975), *J. Chem. Soc. Chem. Comm.*, 290–1.
[70] Murray, M. J. and Hefendehl, F. W. (1973), *Phytochemistry*, **12**, 1875–80.
[71] Yeowell, D. A. and Schmid, H. (1964), *Experientia*, **20**, 250–2.

78   THE BIOSYNTHESIS OF SECONDARY METABOLITES

[72] Cordell, G. A. (1976), *Chem. Rev.*, **76**, 425–60.
[73] Evans, R. and Hanson, J. R. (1976), *J. Chem. Soc. Perkin I*, 326–9.
[74] Milborrow, B. V. (1975), *Phytochemistry*, **14**, 123–8.
[75] Morikawa, K., Hirose, Y. and Nozoe, S. (1971), *Tetrahedron Lett.*, 1131–2.
[76] Ballesia, F., Grandi, R., Marchesini, A., Pagnoni, U. M. and Trave, R. (1975), *Phytochemistry*, **14**, 1737–40.
[77] Croteau, R. and Loomis, W. D. (1972), *Phytochemistry*, **11**, 1055–66.
[78] Souček, M. (1962), *Coll. Czech. Chem. Comm.*, **27**, 2929–33.
[79] Baker, F. C. and Brooks, C. J. W. (1976), *Phytochemistry*, **15**, 689–94.
[80] Overton, K. H. and Picken, D. J. (1976), *J. Chem. Soc. Chem. Comm.*, 105–6.
[81] Birnbaum, G. I., Huber, C. P., Post, M. L., Stothers, J. B., Robinson, J. R., Stoessl, A. and Ward, E. W. B. (1976), *J. Chem. Soc. Chem. Comm.*, 330–1.
[82] Cane, D. E. and Levin, R. H. (1976), *J. Amer. Chem. Soc.*, **98**, 1183–8.
[83] Canonica, L., Kroszczynski, W., Ranzi, B. M., Rindone, B. and Scolastico, C. (1971), *J. Chem. Soc. Chem. Comm.*, 257
[84] Bedford, C. T., Fairlie, J. C., Knittel, P., Money, T. and Phillips, G. T. (1971), *J. Chem. Soc. Chem. Comm.*, pp. 323–4.
[85] Corbella, S., Gariboldi, P., Jommi, G. and Sisti, M. (1975), *J. Chem. Soc. Chem. Comm.*, 288–9.
[86] Biollaz, M. and Arigoni, D. (1969), *J. Chem. Soc. Chem. Comm.*, 633–4.
[87] Corbella, A., Gariboldi, P., Jommi, G. and Scolastico, C. (1969), *J. Chem. Soc. Chem. Comm.*, 634–5.
[88] Edwards, O. E., Douglas, J. L. and Mootoo, B. (1970), *Can. J. Chem.*, **48**, 2517–24.
[89] Dorn, F., Bernasconi, P. and Arigoni, D. (1975), *Chimia (Switz.)*, **29**, 24–5.
[90] Hanson, J. R. and Nyfeler, R. (1975), *J. Chem. Soc. Chem. Comm.*, 824–5.
[91] Tanabe, M., Suzuki, K. T. and Jankowski, W. C. (1974), *Tetrahedron Lett.*, 2271–4.
[92] Hanson, J. R., Marten, T. and Nyfeler, R. (1976), *J. Chem. Soc. Perkin I*, 876–80.
[93] Mellows, G., Mantle, P. G., Feline, T. C. and Williams, D. J. (1973), *Phytochemistry*, **12**, 2717–20.
[94] Hikino, H., Miyase, T. and Takemoto, T. (1976), *Phytochemistry*, **15**, 121–3.
[95] Evans, R., Hanson, J. R. and Marten, T. (1976), *J. Chem. Soc. Perkin I*, 1212–4.
[96] Heinstein, P. F., Herman, D. L., Tove, S. B. and Smith, F. H. (1970), *J. Biol. Chem.*, **245**, 4658–65.
[97] Banerji, A., Jones, R. B., Mellows, G., Phillips, L. and Sim, K.-Y. (1976), *J. Chem. Soc. Perkin. I*, 2221–8.
[98] Banerji, A., Hunter, R., Mellows, G., Sim, K. and Barton, D. H. R. (1978), *J. Chem. Soc. Chem. Comm.*, 843–5.
[99] Adams, M. R. and Bu'Lock, J. D. (1975), *J. Chem. Soc. Chem. Comm.*, 389–91.

[100] Polonsky, J., Lukacs, G., Cagnoli-Bellavita, N. and Ceccherelli, P. (1975), *Tetrahedron Lett.*, 481–4.

[101] Achilladelis, B. and Hanson, J. R. (1969), *J. Chem. Soc. (C)*. 2010–4.

[102] Arigoni, D. (1968), *Pure Appl. Chem.*, **17**, 331–48.

[103] Cross, B. E. (1968), *Progress in Phytochem.*, **1**, 195–222.

[104] Graebe, J. E., Hedden, P. and MacMillan, J. (1975), *J. Chem. Soc. Chem. Comm.*, 161–3.

[105] Dawson, R. M., Jeffries, P. R. and Knox, J. R. (1975), *Phytochemistry*, **14**, 2593–7.

[106] Evans, R. and Hanson, J. R. (1975), *J. Chem. Soc. Perkin I*, 633–6.

[107] Cordell, G. A. (1974), *Phytochemistry*, **13**, 2343–64.

[108] Goodwin, T. W. (1979), *Pure Appl. Chem.*, **51**, 593–6.

[109] Goodwin, T. W. (1972), *Biochem. Soc. Symp.*, **35**, 233–44.

[110] McDermott, J. C. B., Britton, G. and Goodwin, T. W. (1973), *Biochem. J.*, **134**, 1115–7.

[111] Britton, G., Lockley, W. J. S., Patel, N. J., Goodwin, T. W. and Englert, G. (1977), *J. Chem. Soc. Chem. Comm.*, 655–6.

5. The shikimic acid pathway

5.1 Introduction

A compound of unsuspected importance was isolated in 1885 from the fruit of *Illicium religiosum*. To this compound was given the name shikimic acid, a name derived from *shikimi-no-ki* which is the Japanese name for the plant. Shikimic acid (5.7), it transpired from the very elegant studies of much later investigators, is a key intermediate in the biosynthesis of the aromatic amino acids, L-phenylalanine, L-tyrosine and L-tryptophan, in plants and micro-organisms (animals cannot carry out *de novo* synthesis using this pathway). These three aromatic amino acids are individually important precursors for numerous secondary metabolites, and so to some extent are earlier biosynthetic intermediates related to shikimic acid, as the ensuing discussion in this chapter and in Chapters 6 and 7 will show.

Scheme 5.1

80

The biosynthetic pathway through shikimic acid (5.7) to aromatic amino acids, outlined in Scheme 5.1 (acids are shown as anions) is called the shikimic acid or shikimate pathway [1, 2, 5]. It has its origins in carbohydrate metabolism and shows several interesting features, much of it known from detailed examination of the steps involved. The first step is a stereospecific aldol-type condensation between phosphoenolpyruvate (5.1) and D-erythrose-4-phosphate (5.2) to give 3-deoxy-D-arabinoheptulosonic acid 7-phosphate (5.3; DAHP), in which addition occurs to the si-face of the double bond in (5.1) and the re-face of the carbonyl group in (5.2) and which has been rationalized in terms of the mechanism shown in Scheme 5.2

Scheme 5.2

[6]. Ring closure in DAHP (5.3) affords dehydroquinic acid (5.4), which undergoes reversible dehydration to give dehydroshikimic acid (5.6). The addition and elimination of water takes place in an unusual cis sense and has been postulated therefore to occur in a two-step sequence involving an enamine (5.11) formed through the keto-group in (5.4) [7].

(5.11)

Two unexceptional steps lead through shikimic acid (5.7) to its 3-phosphate (5.8). Condensation with phosphoenolpyruvate (5.1) gives (5.9). This type of biological reaction is almost unique, only one other example being known. The mechanism suggested, and illustrated in Scheme 5.3, is based on experiments in deuterium oxide and tritiated water. [The intermediacy of (5.12) is indicated by the random incorporation of hydrogen isotope into the methylene hydrogens of (5.9) [8].]

1,4-Conjugate elimination of phosphoric acid converts (5.9) into chorismic acid (5.10), a reaction which it was shown involves trans elimination of the two groups lost [loss of the (6-pro-R)-hydrogen] [6].

Perhaps the shikimate pathway should be called the chorismate

Scheme 5.3

pathway because it is at chorismic acid (*5.10*) that the single line of biosynthesis fragments into different lines whose termini are the vital aromatic amino acids and diverse other compounds. It appears, however, that the biosynthesis of some microbial metabolites (Section 7.6.1) may divert from the main line at a stage close to shikimic acid (*5.7*)/dehydroquinic acid (*5.4*).

Amination of chorismic acid (*5.10*) leads through anthranilic acid (*5.13*) to tryptophan (*5.14*). The formation of phenylalanine (*5.17*) and tyrosine (*5.18*), on the other hand, proceeds via prephenic acid (*5.16*), whose formation from chorismic acid (*5.10* = *5.15*) involves

(5.13)   (5.14)

(5.15)   (5.16) Prephenic acid   (5.17) R=H, Phenylalanine
                                                 (5.18) R=OH, Tyrosine

what is, formally at least, a Claisen rearrangement—a unique biological example. The same reaction can also be achieved by heating aqueous solutions of chorismic acid (*5.10*), but calculation shows that the enzyme (chorismate mutase) from *Aerobacter aerogenes* enhances the rate of reaction (at pH 7.5 and 37°C) by 1.9×10^6 compared to the purely thermal one. It follows quite reasonably that this is achieved by the enzyme ordering the chorismate molecules into the favoured conformation for reaction [chair transition state, (*5.15*)] and also providing appropriate acid catalysis [8].

† A route from chorismic acid (*5.10*) via isochorismic acid (*5.19*) has been proposed for the biosynthesis of four *m*-carboxy-amino acids,

(5.19) (5.20) (5.21) (5.22)

e.g. (5.20), found in higher plants. Salicylic acid (5.21) also derives from (5.19) [9, 10]. It is interesting to note that aromatization may occur, in micro-organisms, of intermediates of the shikimic acid pathway just after [as for (5.21)] or before chorismic acid (5.10). This leads, for example, to protocatechuic acid (5.22) [11]. Aromatization in this way provides access to phenolic compounds by a route different from those via polyketides (Chapter 3) and, in plants, via aromatic amino acids.

In higher plants the polymer, lignin, and various aromatic secondary metabolites, notably many alkaloids (Chapter 6) and flavonoids (Section 5.4) are formed from the aromatic amino acids, L-phenylalanine (5.17) and/or L-tyrosine (5.18). [For some alkaloids as well as some microbial metabolites, tryptophan (5.14) is the source of their particular aromatic rings.] There are for these metabolites common pathways leading from phenylalanine, and in some plants tyrosine, to phenylpropanoid (C_6-C_3) intermediates. The first step from phenylalanine involves the enzyme L-phenylalanine ammonia lyase (known, perhaps affectionately, as PAL), an enzyme widely distributed, and well-characterized. Elimination of ammonia occurs to give cinnamic acid (5.23). It involves loss of the (3-*pro-S*)-proton of L-phenylalanine (5.17), and thus occurs in the *anti*-sense [L-tyrosine ammonia lyase functions to remove also the (3-*pro-S*)-proton in tyrosine] [12, 13].

p-Coumaric acid (5.24) is the product derived by loss of ammonia from tyrosine (5.18). Much more commonly this acid derives by hydroxylation of cinnamic acid (5.23) formed by ammonia loss from phenylalanine; hydroxylation is accompanied by the usual NIH shift (Section 1.3.2) for this *para*-hydroxylation (also *ortho*-hydroxylation [14]). Up to two further phenolic hydroxy-groups may be introduced on (5.24), Scheme 5.4 [15, 16]. It is interesting to note that in

Phenylalanine
(5.17)

(5.23) Cinnamic acid   (5.24) *p*-Coumaric acid

(5.27) Sinapic acid   (5.26) Ferulic acid   (5.25) Caffeic acid

Scheme 5.4

Mentha species rosmarinic acid (*5.28*) has different origins for its two C_6-C_3 units: independently phenylalanine (*5.17*) for A and tyrosine (*5.18*) for B [17]. [Commonly in higher plants (*5.17*) is not converted into (*5.18*).]

† From the cinnamic acids, (*5.24*)–(*5.27*), β-oxidation and truncation of the side-chains yields a series of benzoic acids [18]. (For gallic acid biosynthesis see [19].) The plant lignins are formed essentially by oxidative polymerization of various cinnamyl alcohols corresponding to the cinnamic acids, (*5.24*), (*5.26*), and (*5.27*) [20]. Three other groups of metabolites, the aryl cyanogenic glucosides, e.g. prunasin (*5.29*) [21], aryl glucosinolates, e.g. (*5.30*) [22] and allylphenols, e.g. eugenol (*5.31*) [23] also derive from phenylalanine. Ferulic acid (*5.26*) is a precursor for both (*5.31*) and [6]-gingerol (*5.32*). The remaining carbon atoms in (*5.32*) derive from a single acetate, with loss of its carboxy-group, and an intact molecule of hexanoic acid [24].

(5.28)   (5.29)   (5.30)

(5.31)   (5.32)

5.2   Quinones [25]

The widely distributed natural quinones are formed by a diversity of routes: several are known for each of the benzoquinones, naphthoquinones and anthraquinones. This can be attributed to the importance which the quinone moiety of these compounds has in the economy of living systems.

The isoprenoid quinones, e.g. the ubiquinones (*5.36*), are essential metabolites, being involved in electron transport in living systems. In the ubiquinones a particular chain length is favoured from $n = 6$ in certain micro-organisms to $n = 10$ in most mammals. Mevalonic acid (*5.33*) is well established as the source of polyprenyl side-chains in these metabolites. It is probable that the side-chain is assembled as a polyprenyl pyrophosphate which then couples with the aromatic fragment. The evidence is that polyprenyl pyrophosphate synthetases and 4-hydroxybenzoate:polyprenyltransferases have been isolated from living systems and ubiquinones co-occur with polyprenyl alcohols [as (*5.34*)] [26, 27].

4-Hydroxybenzoic acid (5.35) has been shown to stand as the key intermediate in ubiquinone biosynthesis, in living systems from micro-organisms to mammals. In animals, phenylalanine and tyrosine serve as precursors, but in bacteria chorismic acid (5.10) is the precursor [28, 29]. Interlocking evidence obtained from bacteria in experiments with mutants (and genetic analysis), cell-free preparations, and isolation and identification of intermediates allows clear delineation [25, 29] of the sequence of biosynthesis as that shown in part in Scheme 5.5; beyond (5.35) the intermediates are the

Scheme 5.5

same in animals and micro-organisms. (In bacteria, at least, it has been concluded that the methoxy-group oxygen derives from molecular oxygen [30].)

The plastoquinones are isoprenoid benzoquinones, (5.40), found in plants and algae which function in photosynthetic electron transport. They include methyl substituents on the quinone ring instead of the methoxy-groups seen in the ubiquinones. Tyrosine (5.18) is the source of the quinone ring [via (5.38) and homogentisic acid (5.39)] but unlike the ubiquinones the side-chain is not lost completely: C-3 is retained as a C-methyl group; the other methyl group derives from methionine (with retention of all three methyl protons). The tyrosine labelling site was deduced by means of a clever degradation sequence [carried out on material biosynthesized from [1,6-^{14}C$_2$]shikimic acid (5.37)]; see Scheme 5.6. The chemical introduction of the third methyl group and Kuhn–Roth (chromic acid–sulphuric acid) oxidation of (5.40) and (5.41) gave a pair of results: ~25% of the total radioactivity in each compound appeared in the acetic acid. This is in accord with the pattern shown (●, ◐); the alternative (■, ◨) would have given acetic containing 25% of the activity of (5.40) and 50% of the activity of (5.41) [31, 32].

† The normal catabolic pathway of tyrosine (5.18) is via 4′–hydroxyphenylpyruvic acid [as (5.38)] and homogenistic acid [as

Scheme 5.6   (5.41)

(5.39)], and is, as we have seen (Scheme 5.6), followed in plasto-quinone formation. A similar course of biosynthesis has been deduced for α- and γ-tocopherol (5.42) and (5.43), respectively (* = methionine derived methyl groups) [31, 32].

(5.42)   (5.43)

†   Helicobasidin (5.45) has been shown to have entirely mevalonoid origins: [2-^{13}C]mevalonate labelled the sites indicated [C-8 and C-10 have become equivalent; only one site will be labelled in the precursor isoprenoid: see (5.44)]. Farnesyl pyrophosphate (5.44) is the appropriate (C$_{15}$) mevalonoid intermediate and in the course of biosynthesis a hydrogen shift (from C-6) occurs, see Scheme 5.7 (cf. Section 4.6) [33, 34].

Scheme 5.7   (5.45) Helicobasidin

The naphthoquinones, exemplified in higher plants by the phyllo-quinones, e.g. vitamin K$_1$ (5.49), and in bacteria by the mena-quinones, e.g. vitamin K$_2$ (5.50), resemble the benzoquinones (above) in structure and function. The polyprenyl side-chains derive from mevalonic acid and the nuclear *C*-methyl groups from methionine. The origin of the remaining atoms is more fascinating.

Experiments with $[1,6\text{-}^{14}C_2]$- and $[3\text{-}^3H]$-shikimic acid establish that the bacterial menaquinones and lawsone *(5.51)*, from the plant *Impatiens balsamina*, derive from shikimate *(5.7)* with C-1 and C-2 appearing at the naphthoquinone ring junction. The carboxy-grou of shikimic acid is retained (at *) on naphthoquinone formation, and *(5.7)* thus accounts for seven of the ten nuclear carbon atoms in e.g. *(5.49)*. [The (6-*pro-S*)-hydrogen is also retained, but the (6-*pro-R*)-proton is lost [35, 36].] The remaining C_3 unit, importantly, was identified as having its origins in glutamic acid or its transamination product, 2-ketoglutaric acid *(5.46)*. Incorporation was of C-2, C-3, and C-4, with loss of C-1 and C-5 [37].

The very efficient incorporation of 2-succinylbenzoate *(5.47)* into plant and bacterial naphthoquinones identifies *(5.47)* as a later

Shikimic acid   *(5.46)*

(5.47)

(5.48)
(i) Oxidation
(ii) prenylation
(iii) methylation

(5.51) Lawsone

(5.49) R =   H, Vitamin K_1
Me   Me $_3$

(5.50)   H ,   Vitamin K_2
Me $_n$

Scheme 5.8 $n = 4, 6, 7$ or 8

intermediate derived from shikimic acid and *(5.46)*. Further corroboration comes from the identification of radioactive *(5.47)* in *I. balsamina* following the feeding of $[U\text{-}^{14}C]$glutamic acid [38, 39]. It appears that diversion from the shikimate pathway to naphthoquinone biosynthesis may occur at chorismic acid *(5.10)* [39]. A plausible mechanism for the formation of 2-succinylbenzoic acid *(5.47)* involving the coenzyme, thiamine pyrophosphate, is shown in Scheme 5.9.

The steps which lie beyond *(5.47)* are not clear but menaquinones and lawsone *(5.51)* are formed from precursors without intervention of a symmetrical intermediate, e.g. 1,4-naphthoquinone *(5.52)*, although the apparently related quinone, juglone *(5.53)*, does derive from this compound [36, 40].

Scheme 5.9

† Other routes have been discovered for naphthoquinone elaboration. The plant quinone, alkannin (5.55), derives from mevalonic
acid (5.33) and the benzoquinone precursor 4-hydroxybenzoic acid
(5.35) (derived in turn from phenylalanine and cinnamic acid). It
seems probable that alkannin is formed via (5.54) [41]. Homogentisic
acid (5.39), the plastoquinone precursor, is a precursor for chimaphi-
lin (5.57), possibly via (5.56). The biosynthesis of naphthoquinones
and benzoquinones from polyketides is found widely in bacteria and
two examples have been identified in plants, plumbagin (5.58) and
7-methyljuglone (5.59) [42]. Anthraquinones may also have polyketide origins [25, 43, 44]. In some cases plant anthraquinones may

derive from 2-succinylbenzoic acid (5.47) e.g. alizarin (5.60) and
morindone (5.61) [45]. The extra carbon atoms derive from a single
unit of mevalonic acid (5.33) as shown in (5.60) and (5.61). The
steps which lie beyond (5.47) are unclear.

$(5.47) \rightarrow (5.48) \longrightarrow$
(5.33)
(5.7) (5.46) (5.33)

(5.60) Alizarin   +   (5.61) Morindone

5.3 Coumarins [46]

† Coumarin (5.63) the simplest of compounds of this type is probably
an artefact arising by enzymatic cleavage of the glucoside (5.62). The
biosynthesis of (5.62)/(5.63) depends crucially on unusual *ortho*-
hydroxylation of cinnamic acid (5.23), and the appropriate enzyme
has been detected [47]. The hydroxycoumarin, umbelliferone (5.64),
arises through *ortho*-hydroxylation of *p*-coumaric acid (5.24). Daphnin
(5.65) and cichorin (5.66) are deduced to derive via umbelliferone
(5.64) [48]. Furanocoumarins, e.g. (5.68), derive from isoprenyl
coumarins [as (5.67)]. The biosynthesis of (5.68) involves (5.64) and
7-demethylsuberosin (5.67) [49, 50] (cf. furoquinoline alkaloid
biosynthesis, Section 6.5).

† Novobiocin (5.69) is produced by a micro-organism, *Streptomyces
niveus*. The origin of the coumarin residue is in tyrosine (and is
thus different from the origins of plant coumarins), and the ring
oxygen derives from the carboxyl oxygen of tyrosine [51].

(5.62)   (5.63) Coumarin   (5.64) Umbelliferone

(5.65) R^1=H, R^2=OH, Daphnin
(5.66) R^1=OH R^2=H, Cichorin

(5.67)   (5.68) Marmesin

(5.69) Novobiocin

5.4 Flavonoids [4]

The flavonoids are found universally in plants as the largest single
group of oxygen ring compounds. They account for a variety of col-
ours found in plant tissues and some, the rotenoids, are insecticidal.
The basic skeleton is found in the flavones, e.g. (5.73); most of the

variations on this pattern are those arising from hydroxylation (and O-methylation and glucoside formation), and oxidation of ring B, as found in the anthocyanidins [as (5.78)]. Some further variation is associated with rearrangement in ring B, found in the isoflavones [as (5.84)], and rotenones [as (5.87)].

Scheme 5.10

The oxygenation pattern shown in (5.73) is characteristic and may be traced back to the origins of the system, namely three acetate units joined head-to-tail (ring A) and a p-coumaryl fragment [as (5.70); rings C and B]. The key stage in the biosynthesis of all flavonoids is reached with the formation of an intermediate chalcone [as (5.71)] ⇌ flavanone [as (5.72)]. Tracer and enzyme evidence points to the formation of chalcones occurring by the condensation of p-coumaryl-coenzyme A with three malonyl-CoA (≃ acetyl-CoA, see Section 3.2.1) units; chalcones are the first identifiable intermediates (Scheme 5.10) [52–54]. The chalcone–flavone interconversion has been shown to be stereospecific as illustrated in Scheme 5.10 [55]. The chalcone, echinatin (5.80), shows an unusual hydroxylation pattern seemingly because the unsaturated ketone function in a normal chalcone has been transposed. This has been shown to be true and transposition occurs of the chalcone (5.79) [56].

(5.79)   (5.80) Echinatin

The hydroxylation pattern of the chalcone is discriminating: those with hydroxy-groups as in (5.71) are converted into 5,7-dihydroxyflavonoids [as (5.73)], those with hydroxy-groups at C-2' and C-4' only [i.e. one oxygen lost from C-6' during chalcone formation, see (5.71)] afford selectively 7-hydroxy-flavonoids [see (5.73)]. The intact incorporation of chalcones into flavonoids has been proved using doubly labelled precursors [57] (for further discussion of this technique see Section 2.2.1).

The weight of evidence from precursor feeding experiments indicates that the extra hydroxy-groups found in ring C, of e.g. quercitin (5.77) are introduced after the chalcone stage of biosynthesis [58]. Moreover, parsley flavone synthase has been found to be highly specific for p-coumaryl-CoA and its single hydroxy-group [54].

It is not yet clear whether the chalcone [as (5.71)] or the flavanone [as (5.72)] is generally involved directly in the formation of flavonoids. Flavones derive from this pair by oxidation. Studies with cell suspension cultures of parsley have given information about the appearance of enzymes involved in the biosynthesis of apiin (5.74) from phenylalanine (5.17). The deduced pathway which proceeds via the flavanone (5.72) is illustrated in Scheme 5.10 [59].

Dihydroflavonols [as (5.75)] are important intermediates in the biosynthesis of other flavonoids. This is illustrated for the biosynthesis of cyanidin (5.78) and quercitin (5.77) in Scheme 5.10; dihydrokaempferol (5.75) was an excellent precursor and its role as an intermediate was confirmed in experiments with a cell culture [60, 61]. In the biosynthesis of taxifolin (5.76) chalcone incorporation was with retention of the C-2 proton [see (5.76)]. This excludes a flavone intermediate and formation of (5.76) can very reasonably be thought to occur via the epoxide (5.81) [62].

(5.81)   Taxifolin (5.76)

The formation of isoflavonoids, e.g. formononetin (5.84), is proved to occur by rearrangement of the chalcone skeleton involving a 1,2-aryl shift. A possible mechanism which leads alternatively to aurones [as (5.82)] is illustrated in Scheme 5.11. Coumestrol (5.86) and

Scheme 5.11

(5.82)

(5.83) R = H
(5.84) R = Me, Formononetin

rotenone (5.87) derive also by a 1,2-aryl shift within a chalcone pre-cursor [63–67]: the chalcone [(5.85); ^{14}C label: ●] gave coumestrol [(5.86); label as shown]; the phenylalanine labelling of rotenone [(5.87); ●, ▲: ^{14}C] is shown. Careful work has allowed detailed delineation of amorphigenin (5.88) biosynthesis [68]. The extra ring carbon atom in these rotenoids derives (oxidatively) from a methoxy-group and for amorphigenin (5.88) the substrate for forma-tion of the additional ring is (5.89).

(5.85)

(5.86) Coumestrol

Phenylalanine

(5.87) R = Me, Rotenone
(5.88) R = CH$_2$OH, Amorphigenin

(5.89)

† Calophyllolide (5.90) is one of a group of neoflavonoids which can be thought of as arising from the same basic units as other flavonoids but in a different manner (Scheme 5.12). In accord with this, label from [3-^{14}C]phenylalanine [as (5.17)] was found to be located as shown in (5.90) (●: ^{14}C label) [69].

† Stilbenes, e.g. oxyresveratrol (5.92), have been found to occur throughout the plant kingdom. A pathway to them analogous to that

Scheme 5.12

(5.90) Calophyllolide

(5.91)

(5.92) Oxyresveratrol

Scheme 5.13

for chalcone formation (Scheme 5.13) i.e. via (5.91), is indicated by the pattern of acetate and cinnamate incorporation shown [70, 71].

References

Further reading: [1]–[4].

[1] Haslam, E. (1979), in *Comprehensive Organic Chemistry* (eds. D. H. R. Barton and W. D. Ollis), Pergamon, Oxford, vol. 5, pp. 1167–205.

[2] Haslam, E. (1974), *The Shikimate Pathway*, Butterworths, London.

[3] *Biosynthesis*, (*Specialist Periodical Reports*) [ed. T. A. Geissman (vols. 1–3), J. D. Bu'Lock (vols. 4 and 5)], The Chemical Society, London.

[4] Hahlbrock, K. and Grisebach, H. (1975), in *The Flavonoids* (eds. J. B. Harborne, T. J. Mabry and H. Mabry), Chapman and Hall, London, pp. 866–915.

[5] Gibson, F. and Pittard, J. (1968), *Bact. Rev.*, **32**, 465–92.

[6] Floss, H. G., Onderka, D. K. and Carroll, M. (1972), *J. Biol. Chem.*, **247**, 736–44.

[7] Turner, M. J., Smith, B. W. and Haslam, E. (1975), *J. Chem. Soc. Perkin I*, 52–5.

[8] Ife, R., Ball, L. F., Lowe, P. and Haslam, E. (1976), *J. Chem. Soc. Perkin I*, 1776–83.

[9] Larsen, P. O. and Wieczorkowska, E. (1975), *Biochim. Biophys. Acta*, **381**, 409–15.

[10] Marshall, B. J. and Ratledge, C. (1972), *Biochim. Biophys. Acta*, **264**, 106–16.

[11] Scharf, K. H., Zenk, M. H., Onderka, D. K., Carroll, M. and Floss, H. G. (1971), *J. Chem. Soc. Chem. Comm.*, 765–6.

[12] Camm, E. L. and Towers, G. H. N. (1973), *Phytochemistry*, **12**, 961–73.

[13] Strange, P. G., Staunton, J., Wiltshire, H. R., Battersby, A. R., Hanson, K. R. and Havir, E. A. (1972), *J. Chem. Soc. Perkin I*, 2364–72.

[14] Ellis, B. E. and Amrhein, N. (1971), *Phytochemistry*, **10**, 3069–72.

[15] Amrhein, N. and Zenk, M. H. (1969), *Phytochemistry*, **8**, 107–13.

[16] Neish, A. C. (1964), in *Biochemistry of Phenolic Compounds* (ed. J. B. Harborne), Academic Press, New York, pp. 294–359.

[17] Ellis, B. E. and Towers, G. H. N. (1970), *Biochem. J.*, **118**, 291–7.

[18] Zenk, M. H. (1966), in *Biosynthesis of Aromatic Compounds* (ed. G. Billek), Pergamon, pp. 45–60.

[19] Dewick, P. M. and Haslam, E. (1969), *Biochem. J.*, **113**, 537–42.

[20] Higuchi, T. (1971), *Adv. Enzymol.*, **34**, 207–83.

[21] Tapper, B. A., Zilg, H. and Conn, E. E. (1972), *Phytochemistry*, **11**, 1047–53.

[22] Matsuo, M., Kirkland, D. F. and Underhill, E. W. (1972), *Phytochemistry*, **11**, 697–701.

[23] Klischies, M., Stöckigt, J. and Zenk, M. H. (1975), *J. Chem. Soc. Chem. Comm.*, 879–80.

[24] Denniff, P. and Whiting, D. A. (1976), *J. Chem. Soc. Chem. Comm.*, 711–2.

[25] Bentley, R. (1975), in *Biosynthesis (Specialist Periodical Reports)* (ed. T. A. Geissman), The Chemical Society, London, vol. 3, pp. 181–246.

[26] Allen, C. M., Alworth, W., MacRae, A. and Bloch, K. (1967), *J. Biol. Chem.*, **242**, 1895–902.

[27] Hemming, F. W., Morton, R. A. and Pennock, J. F. (1963), *Proc. Roy. Soc.*, **158B**, 291–310.

[28] Olson, R. E. (1966), *Vitam. Horm.*, **24**, 551–74.

[29] Young, I. G., Stroobant, P., MacDonald, C. G. and Gibson, F. (1973), *J. Bacteriol.*, **114**, 42–52.

[30] Uchida, K. and Aida, K. (1972), *Biochem. Biophys. Res. Comm.*, **46**, 130–5.

[31] Threlfall, D. R. (1972), *Biochim. Biophys. Acta*, **280**, 472–80.

[32] Whistance, G. R. and Threlfall, D. R. (1971), *Phytochemistry*, **10**, 1533–8.

[33] Adams, P. M. and Hanson, J. R. (1972), *J. Chem. Soc. Perkin I*, 586–8.

[34] Tanabe, M., Suzuki, K. T. and Jankowski, W. C. (1973), *Tetrahedron Lett.*, 4723–6.

[35] Baldwin, R. M., Snyder, C. D. and Rapoport, H. (1973), *J. Amer. Chem. Soc.*, **95**, 276–8.

[36] Scharf, K.-H., Zenk, M. H., Onderka, D. K., Carroll, M. and Floss, H. G. (1971), *J. Chem. Soc. Chem. Comm.*, 576–7.

[37] Campbell, I. M., Robins, D. J., Kelsey, M. and Bentley, R. (1971), *Biochemistry*, **10**, 3069–78.

[38] Grotzinger, E. and Campbell, I. M. (1974), *Phytochemistry*, **13**, 923–6.

[39] Dansette, P. and Azerad, R. (1970), *Biochem. Biophys. Res. Comm.*, **40**, 1090–5.

[40] Grotzinger, E. and Campbell, I. M. (1972), *Phytochemistry*, **11**, 675–9.

[41] Schmid, H. V. and Zenk, M. H. (1971), *Tetrahedron Lett.*, 4151–5.

[42] Durand, R. and Zenk, M. H. (1971), *Tetrahedron Lett.*, 3009–12.

[43] Steglich, W., Arnold, R., Lösel, W. and Reiniger, W. (1972), *J. Chem. Soc. Chem. Comm.*, 102–3.

[44] Curtis, R. F., Hassall, C. H. and Parry, D. R. (1971), *J. Chem. Soc. Chem. Comm.*, 410.

[45] Leistner, E. (1973), *Phytochemistry*, **12**, 1669–74.

THE SHIKIMIC ACID PATHWAY 95

[46] Brown, S. A. (1966), in *Biosynthesis of Aromatic Compounds* (ed. G. Billek), Pergamon, pp. 15–24.
[47] Gestetner, B. and Conn, E. E. (1974), *Arch. Biochem. Biophys.*, **163**, 617–24.
[48] Satô, M. and Hasegawa, M. (1972), *Phytochemistry*, **11**, 657–62.
[49] Austin, D. J. and Brown, S. A. (1973), *Phytochemistry*, **12**, 1657–67.
[50] Brown, S. A. and Steck, W. (1973), *Phytochemistry*, **12**, pp. 1315–24.
[51] Bunton, C. A., Kenner, G. W., Robinson, M. J. T. and Webster, B. R. (1963), *Tetrahedron*, **19**, 1001–10.
[52] Grisebach, H. and Barz, W. (1969), *Naturwiss.*, **56**, 538–44.
[53] Grisebach, H. (1968), in *Recent Advances in Phytochemistry*, **1**, 379–406.
[54] Hrazdina, G., Kreuzaler, F., Hahlbrock, K. and Grisebach, H. (1976), *Arch. Biochem. Biophys.*, **175**, 392–9.
[55] Hahlbrock, K., Zilg, H. and Grisebach, H. (1970), *Eur. J. Biochem.*, **15**, 13–18.
[56] Saitoh, T., Shibata, S., Sankawa, U., Furuya, T. and Ayabe, S. (1975), *Tetrahedron Lett.*, 4463–6.
[57] Patschke, L., Grisebach, H. and Barz, W. (1964), *Z. Naturforsch.*, **19b**, 1110–3.
[58] Patschke, L. and Grisebach, H. (1965), *Z. Naturforsch.*, **20b**, 1039–42.
[59] Hahlbrock, K., Ebel, J., Ortmann, R., Sutter, A., Wellmann, E. and Grisebach, H. (1971), *Biochim. Biophys. Acta*, **244**, 7–15.
[60] Fritsch, H., Hahlbrock, K. and Grisebach, H. (1971), *Z. Naturforsch.*, **26b**, 581–5.
[61] Fritsch, H. and Grisebach, H. (1975), *Phytochemistry*, **14**, 2437–41.
[62] Grisebach, H. and Kellner, S. (1965), *Z. Naturforsch.*, **20b**, 446–50.
[63] Pelter, A., Bradshaw, J. and Warren, R. F. (1971), *Phytochemistry*, **10**, 835–50.
[64] Wong, E. (1968), *J. Chem. Soc. Chem. Comm.*, 395.
[65] Dewick, P. M. (1977), *Phytochemistry*, **16**, 93–7.
[66] Grisebach, H. and Barz, W. (1964), *Z. Naturforsch.*, **19b**, 569–71.
[67] Berlin, J., Dewick, P. M., Barz, W. and Grisebach, H. (1972), *Phytochemistry*, **11**, 1689–93.
[68] Crombie, L., Dewick, P. M. and Whiting, D. A. (1971), *J. Chem. Soc. Chem. Comm.*, 1183–5.
[69] Kunesch, G. and Polonsky, J. (1969), *Phytochemistry*, **8**, 1221–6.
[70] Billek G. and Schimpl, A. (1966), in *Biosynthesis of Aromatic Compounds* (ed. G. Billek), Pergamon, pp. 37–44.
[71] Billek, G. and Schimpl, A. (1962), *Monatshefte*, **93**, 1457–9.

6. Alkaloids

6.1 Introduction

Basic nitrogenous metabolites isolated from plants are called alkaloids. There are very many of them, and they have diverse structures [1, 2]. Yet an examination of these structures indicates that alkaloids can be classified within a few groups, as will be apparent from the discussion below. This is because they are formed very largely from a handful of α-amino acids, lysine, ornithine, phenylalanine, tyrosine and tryptophan, and the skeletons of these amino acids are retained largely intact in the derived alkaloids. Mevalonate and acetate are further important starting points from primary metabolism.

Economy in the use of a few primary metabolites has been of importance in allowing the development of useful ideas [3] about alkaloid biosynthesis, e.g. tropine (6.3) and hygrine (6.2) could be thought of simply as deriving from ornithine and acetate (see Scheme 6.1). Two further things have been important in useful speculation

Scheme 6.1

about alkaloid biosynthesis: (i) structures of similar alkaloids often suggest plausible biosynthetic relationships, e.g. hygrine (6.2), formed in the same species as esters of (6.3), might well be an intermediate in the formation of tropine (6.3); (ii) alkaloid formation involves simple, almost repetitive, reactions, and, most widely, those of the type summarized in Scheme 6.2. Such a reaction is proposed for the formation of hygrine (6.2) and is one that can be carried out in the laboratory (see Scheme 6.3 and Section 6.2.2).

Scheme 6.2

96

Scheme 6.3

Another, crucially important, reaction type, encountered in the biosynthesis of aromatic alkaloids, is the joining together of benzene rings which is thought to occur by what is called phenol oxidative coupling (for further discussion see Section 1.3.1).

In the living plant, the roles (and there is surely not just one role) that alkaloids have to play are largely obscure, but it is to be noted that plants tend to synthesize alkaloids of similar structure some-times by different pathways (see e.g. Section 6.2.1). Clearly, particu-lar structural types are (or have been) important to the survival of at least some plants.

6.2   Piperidine and pyrrolidine alkaloids

6.2.1   Piperidine alkaloids

Simple examples of piperidine alkaloids are N-methylpelletierine (6.19) and the hemlock alkaloid, coniine (6.14). In these bases the structural relationship is manifestly close. This relationship is similarly apparent between anabasine (6.20) and anatabine (6.7) which are, moreover, found in the same plant. It is however, clear, from biosynthetic experiments, that whilst the piperidine rings of N-methylpelletierine (6.19) and anabasine (6.20) derive from the amino acid lysine (6.17) those of coniine (6.14) and, most surprisingly, anatabine (6.7) have quite different origins. It is proved that anatabine (6.7) is formed from two molecules of nicotinic acid (6.4) [4] (the labelling results, and a suggested pathway, is illustrated in Scheme 6.4). Only the pyridine ring of anabasine derives from

Scheme 6.4

nicotinic acid (*6.4*). For both alkaloids, however, the point of attachment of ring A is C-3, the site of the carboxy-group in (*6.5*). Presumably this group assists in the condensation between the two heterocycles in the course of the biosynthesis of each alkaloid (see Scheme 6.4, cf. Scheme 6.15). For evidence on the likely intermediacy of (*6.5*) in the biosynthesis of the analogous base, nicotine, see Section 6.2.2.

Dioscorine (*6.8*) is, like anatabine, exceptional in that the piperidine ring (heavy bonding) also derives from nicotinic acid (*6.4*); the remaining atoms derive from acetate (acetoacetate) [see (*6.9*)] [5].

The entire skeleton of coniine (*6.14*) derives from acetate, with labelling of C-2', C-2, C-4, and C-6 by [1-^{14}C]acetate. A polyketide pathway immediately seems likely and 5-oxo-octanoic acid (*6.11*) and the corresponding aldehyde (*6.12*), with the necessary functionality for inclusion of the nitrogen atom, were shown, by tracer and enzymic evidence, to be implicated in coniine biosynthesis, as was γ-coniceine (*6.13*) which is also a hemlock alkaloid. These results [6, 7] lead in a straightforward way to the pathway shown in Scheme 6.5. Most curiously, however, it has been found that octanoic acid

Scheme 6.5

(*6.10*) is a significant and specific precursor for coniine (*6.14*). It follows from this that coniine may be formed oxidatively from a C-8 fatty acid, (*6.10*), rather than reductively from a C-8 polyketide. If this is so, then this alkaloid is almost unique in the field of secondary metabolism since very few other acetate-derived metabolites so far investigated are known to arise through fatty acids.

Pinidine (*6.15*) [8], with a structure similar to that of coniine (*6.14*), also derives by simple linear combination of acetate units: C-2, C-4, C-6, and C-9 were labelled by [1-^{14}C]acetate. One of the acetate carboxy groups is lost during biosynthesis (from C-1 or C-10). Non-radioactive sodium acetate fed at the same time as diethyl [1-^{14}C]malonate diluted radioactivity from C-2 which must therefore be part of the 'starter' acetate unit (see Chapter 3), i.e. the carboxy group is lost from C-10. This, in the light of coniine biosynthesis, leads to (*6.16*), and possibly decanoic acid, as intermediates

(6.15) Pinidine   (6.16)

in pinidine formation but so far negative results have been obtained in feeding experiments with these compounds.

The pathways deduced for coniine (6.14) and pinidine (6.15) on the one hand, and anatabine (6.7) and dioscorine (6.8) on the other, are exceptional. That deduced for N-methylpelletierine (6.19) can be considered much more typical of piperidine alkaloids because the piperidine ring originates from lysine (6.17). Two other alkaloids, anabasine (6.20) and sedamine (6.21) have similar origins and much of the evidence for the three alkaloids is interlocking so they are best discussed together.

(6.17) Lysine   (6.18) Δ¹-Piperideine   (6.19) N-Methylpelletierine

(6.20) Anabasine   Scheme 6.6   (6.21) Sedamine

The results of extensive experiments with variously labelled samples of lysine closely define the way in which this amino acid is assimilated into the alkaloids. Thus C-2 and C-6 of the precursor become C-2 and C-6, respectively, in (6.19) [9], (6.21) [10, 11], and (6.20) [12]. Although cadaverine (6.26) is also an alkaloid precursor it cannot be an intermediate *following* lysine because any label at C-2 or C-6 of the amino acid would become spread over both C-1 and C-5 of the symmetrical diamine (6.26); a single lysine label would thus be spread over both C-2 and C-6 of the alkaloids.

Tritium at C-2 and C-6 of lysine is retained on formation of sedamine (6.21) [10, 11]. These results, supported by those with [¹⁵N]-labelled samples of lysine, indicate that alkaloid formation involves retention of the C-6 amino-group and loss of the one at C-2. Loss of the C-6 amino group would require oxidation of C-6 and tritium loss, but removal of the other amino-group is not expected, necessarily, to result in tritium loss from C-2. The reaction may be one of deaminative decarboxylation (see below) leading to Δ¹-

piperideine (*6.18*); [6-^{14}C]-labelled (*6.18*) was specifically incorporated into anabasine (*6.20*) with labelling of C-6 [13].

The origins of the skeletal fragments of (*6.19*), (*6.20*), and (*6.21*) not accounted for by lysine (and Δ^1-piperideine) are as follows. The C$_3$ side-chain in *N*-methylpelletierine (*6.19*) has its origins in acetate plausibly via acetoacetate [9]. The side-chain of sedamine (*6.21*), on the other hand, derives from phenylalanine, probably by way of its deamination product, cinnamic acid [10, 11]. Benzoylacetic acid, a normal *in vivo* transformation product of cinnamic acid, may also reasonably be included in the pathway to this alkaloid, as it is in, e.g., the biosynthesis of lobeline (*6.34*) and of phenanthroindolizidine alkaloids (see Section 6.2.2). The pyridine ring of anabasine (*6.20*) arises from nicotinic acid [14] by way presumably of (*6.5*) (cf. nicotine, Section 6.2.2). The acid precursors (see Scheme 6.6) for (*6.19*), (*6.20*) and (*6.21*), have in common an electron-donating functionality (Scheme 6.7) which may react with Δ^1-piperideine (*6.18*), possibly with concommitant decarboxylation, to give the alkaloids (cf. fatty acid biosynthesis, Section 1.1.2).

Scheme 6.7

In the case of sedamine (*6.21*) and *N*-methylpelletierine (*6.19*) a further step of methylation is required and it was at one time thought that the incorporation of lysine with distinction between C-2 and C-6, as well as the incorporation of cadaverine (*6.26*), could be accommodated in terms of ε-*N*-methyl-lysine [see (*6.17*)], *N*-methylcadaverine (*6.24*) and *N*-methyl-Δ^1-piperideine (*6.22*). However, it has been shown that (*6.22*) is not implicated in anabasine (*6.20*) biosynthesis but does afford *in vivo* the unnatural base (*6.23*) [15], and that *N*-methylcadaverine (*6.24*) is not present in plants

(*6.22*)   (*6.23*)   (*6.24*)

producing (*6.21*) (*Sedum* species) and (*6.20*). Most importantly it has been shown [16] that although ε-*N*-methyl-lysine [see (*6.17*)] is a natural constituent of *Sedum acre*, it was formed from [6-^{3}H]lysine and [*Me*-^{14}C]methionine (source of the *N*-methyl groups) with an isotope ratio which differed from that of sedamine (*6.21*) formed in the same experiment, clearly excluding a precursor–product relationship between the two compounds.

A brilliantly simple and largely satisfying solution [16] to the observations on lysine and cadaverine incorporation has been proposed. It is consistent in particular with the observed incorporation of lysine with distinction between C-2 and C-6, loss of nitrogen from C-2 but retention of the C-2 proton and it allows for normal incorporation of cadaverine (6.26). Central to the proposal is enzyme-catalysed decarboxylation of lysine (lysine decarboxylase) and oxidation of cadaverine (diamine oxidase) both involving pyridoxal phosphate as coenzyme. The proposed sequence involves orthodox pyridoxal-linked intermediates of which (6.25) and (6.27) are common to both enzyme-mediated reactions (Scheme 6.8). It is an important

Scheme 6.8

point that the cadaverine formed from lysine remains coenzyme-bound to preserve the distinction between C-2 and C-6. There are some alkaloids, as we shall see, where this distinction is lost, and it is suggested that only in these cases does equilibration of bound with unbound cadaverine occur.

On the basis of the above hypothesis, cadaverine (6.26) assumed importance as a normal precursor for piperidine alkaloids, and it has been shown that its incorporation into N-methylpelletierine (6.19) involves stereospecific loss of one of the C-1 protons [the (pro-S)-hydrogen atom] [17]; this is accommodated within the model sequence. Decarboxylation of the lysine is also stereospecific (for the L, or S, isomer), but curiously the results indicate apparently that protonation of (6.25) in plants proceeds with opposite stereochemistry to that observed in micro-organisms [18].

In contrast to alkaloid formation which is preferentially from L-lysine, the genesis of pipecolic acid (6.28), which is found widely in plants, animals and micro-organisms, is preferentially from D-lysine [19, 20]. Significantly the biosynthetic pathway to pipecolic acid, illustrated in Scheme 6.9, is different from that which leads to piperidine alkaloids (Scheme 6.8) [11].

Scheme 6.9   (6.28) Pipecolic acid

The unit (6.29) found in sedamine (6.21) and N-methylpelletierine (6.19) is one which occurs widely in piperidine alkaloids, a number of which have had their biosynthesis investigated, and proved to be largely as expected: anaferine (6.31) [9] and pseudopelletierine (6.32) [16] (for a full discussion on related pyrrolidine alkaloids see Section 6.2.2), (6.33) [21], lobeline (6.34) [22], (6.35) [22] and also lobinaline (6.36) which is formed from two molecules of 2-phenacylpiperidine (6.30) (see dotted line) [23]. Securinine (6.37) [24, 25] is manifestly not

(6.29)
(6.30) R = Ph

(6.31)

(6.32)

(6.33)

(6.34)

(6.35)

(6.36)

Δ¹ Piperideine

Tyrosine

(6.37) Securinine

composed from the (6.29) unit. Carbons 6–13 derive from the aromatic amino acid tyrosine, in a pathway for which no analogies can as yet be seen. It is clear, however, that at some stage condensation occurs with Δ¹-piperideine, since both it, lysine, and cadaverine are specific precursors for the piperidine ring of securinine (6.37) in the expected manner; label from C-2 of the first two precursors appears at C-5 of the alkaloid, thus defining the orientation of the Δ¹-piperideine double bond as that shown. It is interesting to note, from these results, that incorporation of lysine avoids a symmetrical intermediate and it is so far the only base with a nitrogen atom common to two rings which does so (see the discussion of Lythraceae and Lycopodium alkaloids below).

Experience with the biosynthetic pathways to anatabine (6.7) and anabasine (6.20) does not allow us to predict with security the likely origins of adenocarpine (6.39) and santiaguine (6.41). Indeed, here lysine is the progenitor for all four nitrogen heterocycles in santiaguine; incorporation is without intervention of a symmetrical intermediate (see Scheme 6.10). Biosynthesis has been shown [26] to

(6.41) Santiaguine   Scheme 6.10

proceed from lysine through Δ^1-piperideine (6.18) and its dimer (6.38) to adenocarpine (6.39) and thence to santiaguine (6.41). This alkaloid arises then by a $2\pi + 2\pi$ dimerization of adenocarpine, although an alternative, if apparently less important, route involves combination of truxillic acid (6.40) with (6.38); (6.40) itself arises from phenylalanine via cinnamic acid. Concerted chemical $2\pi + 2\pi$ dimerization is photochemically mediated, but interestingly occurs in vivo whether the plants are in light or dark.

The biosynthesis of the structurally complex alkaloids of the primitive club moss (Lycopodium species), e.g. lycopodine (6.43) and cernuine (6.44), has been analysed simply in terms of a pathway which involves the dimerization of two pelletierine units (Scheme 6.11). Substance is given to this hypothesis by the appropriate incorporations of acetate, lysine (6.17), and Δ^1-piperideine (6.18) into lycopodine (6.43) and cernuine (6.44). Significantly, these precursors were incorporated equally into both putative pelletierine (C_8N) units [27].

The crucial test for the hypothesis lay with the examination of pelletierine (6.42) as a precursor. The results were quite unexpected for, although pelletierine (6.42) was incorporated as an intact unit, it labelled only one of the C_8N units (shown with heavy bonding) in lycopodine (6.43) and cernuine (6.44). It was subsequently shown that pelletierine (6.42) is a normal constituent of the plant used to

(6.42) Pelletierine   *(6.43)* Lycopodine

Scheme 6.11   *(6.44)* Cernuine

study lycopodine biosynthesis and is formed from lycopodine precursors. Unlabelled pelletierine, when fed with radioactive cadaverine or Δ^1-piperideine, very efficiently diluted activity in the one C_8N unit (heavy bonding) of lycopodine *(6.43)* for which it is a precursor. It follows that pelletierine is a normal intermediate in the biosynthesis of lycopodine (and cernuine), but unlike the other precursors tested is involved in the biosynthesis of only one unit. The equal labelling of both C_8N units by Δ^1-piperideine *(6.18)* (and lysine) requires that the second C_8N unit must be closely related to pelletierine *(6.42)*: significant differences in structure would be associated with differing pathways and hence unequal incorporation of label into the two C_8N units. The results argue thus for the pelletierine-dimer hypothesis, but in modified form. It is not easy, however, to propose modifications to the pathway which will fit the results. Hypotheses surrounding *(6.45)* and *(6.46)* as intermediates have not been supported by subsequent experimentation. So the puzzle remains. One possibility not so far examined is *(6.47)*, potentially an intermediate in the condensation of *(6.18)* with acetoacetate (cf. Scheme 6.7).

(6.45)   *(6.46)*   *(6.47)*

Both the *Lycopodium* [27] and Lythraceae [28, 29] alkaloids, e.g. decodine *(6.49)* and cryogenine *(6.48)* derive from lysine in such a way that C-2 and C-6 become equivalent, logically via cadaverine *(6.26)* (cf. Scheme 6.8). This contrasts with the other piperidine alkaloids discussed above.

The labelling sites of decodine *(6.49)* and decinine *(6.50)* formed from [2-^{14}C]lysine [as *(6.17)*] were C-5 and C-9. This locates ring A as being derived from this amino acid. Ring D plus attached C_3 unit [see especially *(6.48)*] corresponds to a cinnamic acid derivative, and it has been shown that this fragment derives from phenylalanine, a

(6.51) Phenylalanine

(6.48) R^1 = H R^2 = OMe, $\Delta^{1'}$, Cryogenine
(6.49) R^1 = OH, R^2 = H, Decodine
(6.50) R^1 = H, R^2 = OMe, Decinine

known precursor for cinnamic acid: $[1,3\text{-}^{14}C_2]$phenylalanine labelled C-1′, C-3′, and C-1 of decodine (6.49). The labelling of C-1 shows that the amino acid is the source too of ring D plus C-1 but not C-3. The results cannot say whether C-2 derives from phenylalanine but if one considers the genesis of the remaining atoms, pelletierine (6.42) is a likely intermediate. So acetate (acetoacetate) probably accounts for C-2, C-3, and C-4, with the acetoacetate oxygen still present at C-3 forming one point of attachment for the macrocyclic ring, the other, between rings C and D, arising by oxidative phenolic coupling (Section 1.3.1).

Lupinine (6.52) is one representative of a group of quinolizidine alkaloids which includes bases (6.53) through (6.58). It is structurally one of the simplest. Slightly more complex is sparteine (6.53) which like lupinine is a major alkaloid of the bitter form of the yellow lupin. Specific incorporation of cadaverine in the manner shown (Scheme 6.12) indicates an origin for both exclusively in cadaverine with two and three molecules being involved. $[2\text{-}^{14}C]$Lysine labelled the same sites, so, as with other alkaloids having nitrogen common to two rings (except securinine), incorporation is through a symmetrical intermediate [30, 31]. Further evidence indicates firmly that lysine incorporation is by way of the symmetrical base, cadaverine [32].

Lysine (6.17)

Cadaverine

(6.52) Lupinine   (6.53) Sparteine

Scheme 6.12

The implied relationship between lupinine (6.52) and sparteine (6.53) is given substance by the observation that the bicyclic base is the precursor for the tetracyclic one [33]. Results of experiments with $^{14}CO_2$ indicate that sparteine (6.53) and lupanine (6.54) have a partially independent biogenesis. The latter serves as a precursor via its 5,6-dehydro-derivative for bases with a pyridone ring, e.g. thermopsine (6.55) [34, 35]. Since radioactivity from $^{14}CO_2$ appeared in tet-

(6.54) Lupanine

(6.55) Thermopsine

(6.56) Rhombifoline

(6.57) Cytisine

(6.58) Matrine

(6.59)

racyclic bases before the tricyclic ones, e.g. (6.56) and (6.57), it follows that the tricyclic skeleton is formed by fragmentation of the tetracyclic one. It seems, moreover, that rhombifoline (6.56) plays a primary role in the formation of cytisine (6.57).

An alternative tetracyclic skeleton to the one found in sparteine (6.53) is seen in matrine (6.58) and a similar derivation from three molecules of lysine via cadaverine has been demonstrated ($\bullet$ = ^{14}C labels, as in Scheme 6.12) [36, 37].

Little secure information exists on the detail of biosynthesis between cadaverine and the various alkaloids although the incorporation, in appropriate fashion, of three molecules of radioactive Δ^1-piperideine (6.18) into lupanine (6.54) has been recorded: label from C-6 appeared at C-2, C-15, and, by inference, C-10, whereas C-2 label appeared at C-17, C-11, and, by inference, C-6 [38]. (Much less definitive results were obtained for matrine [36].) This was taken, together with a careful consideration of the chirality at the asymmetric centres of all the quinolizidine alkaloids, as evidence for rearrangement within the Δ^1-piperideine trimer (6.59) [38], formed from (6.18), leading to the quinolizidine alkaloids [38].

6.2.2   Pyrrolidine alkaloids

Reactions which occur under so-called 'physiological conditions', i.e. in aqueous solution at pH 7 and room temperature, can provide a reliable guide to actual biological reactions. Thus the condensation of acetoacetic acid with N-methyl-Δ^1-pyrroline (6.64) to give the naturally occurring alkaloid hygrine (6.2) [39], is also most probably the same reaction which occurs *in vivo* (see Scheme 6.3); a more complex example is given later in this section when discussing the biosynthesis of phenanthroindolizidine alkaloids and there are many more most notably in the area of terpenoid indole alkaloids (Section 6.6.2).

On the other hand, the classical and spectacular synthesis of tropinone (6.65) by reaction of succindialdehyde, methylamine and

Scheme 6.13

acetonedicarboxylic acid under 'physiological conditions' is a quite misleading guide to the biosynthesis of the group of tropane alkaloids, exemplified by hyoscyamine (6.67) [40]. They are formed instead from the amino acid ornithine (6.60) (incorporation of [2-^{14}C]-labelled material) [41, 42] and putrescine (6.63) is also implicated. Label from [1,4-^{14}C$_2$]putrescine was confined to the bridgehead carbons of e.g. hyoscyamine (6.67) [43]. Equal labelling of the bridgehead carbons by putrescine is expected, but the single label from [2-^{14}C]ornithine, whilst it should be located at the bridgehead, might appear at one or both of the bridgehead atoms (cf. the discussion of the analogous situation in the formation of piperidine alkaloids from lysine, Section 6.2.1). An ingenious and elegant degradative sequence was developed which established the ornithine labelling pattern [41]. The labelled hyoscyamine (6.69) was converted into the racemate (6.70) (see Scheme 6.14) which was resolved. Further degradation allowed isolation of the carbon atom to which the amino-group, in each enantiomer, was attached. These

Scheme 6.14

carbon atoms correspond to the two bridgehead atoms in (6.69) and a distinction between them was thus achieved.

It was found that [2-^{14}C]ornithine labelled only one of the bridge-head positions. It follows from this that the incorporation of the amino acid is unsymmetrical and cannot therefore involve the symmetrical base putrescine as an intermediate. As a result of corroborating tracer experiments obtained for tropane alkaloids and cuscohygrine (6.68), it is currently believed [44] that unsymmetrical ornithine incorporation is achieved through methylation to N-methylornithine (6.61) followed by decarboxylation to give N-methylputrescine (6.62); this latter unsymmetrical base may also be formed from putrescine (6.63). It is to be noted that this pathway differs from that deduced for piperidine alkaloids, where non-symmetrical incorporation of the precursor amino acid (lysine) is more simply accounted for (Section 6.2.1).

In the biosynthesis of nicotine (6.71) in *Nicotiana* species it has been found [45, 46] that both ornithine (6.60) and putrescine (6.63) are again involved in pyrrolidine-ring formation. For this alkaloid, however, incorporation of the amino acid is through at least one symmetrical intermediate, logically putrescine (6.63), because [2-^{14}C]ornithine gave nicotine (6.71) with label equally spread over C-2' and C-5'; additional results were obtained with [^{15}N]ornithines. This symmetrical pathway is supported by experiments with $^{14}CO_2$, although a few results indicate an unsymmetrical route [47, 48].

Scheme 6.15

The intact incorporations into nicotine (6.71) of N-methylputrescine (6.62) and N-methyl-Δ^1-pyrroline (6.64) further define the pathway to this alkaloid [significantly label from C-2 of the precursor (6.64) appeared at C-2' of the alkaloid]. N-Methyl-Δ^1-pyrroline (6.64) was isolated in radioactive form after feeding, for example, radioactive ornithine to *Nicotiana* species, thus establishing its role as an intermediate in nicotine biosynthesis. Additional persuasive evidence comes from the isolation from *Nicotiana* of an enzyme which catalyses the conversion of putrescine

(6.63) into (6.62), and one which effects the transformation of (6.62) into (6.64) [49].

The pyridine ring of nicotine has been proved to have its genesis in nicotinic acid (6.4) and the pyrrolidine ring becomes attached to the site from which the carboxy group is lost. The mechanism whereby the two rings join is suggested by the results obtained with deuteriated and tritiated nicotinic acid samples: hydrogen isotope appears to be lost from C-6, and C-6 only. This is not the result of hydroxylation at this site because 6-hydroxynicotinic acid is not a nicotine precursor. Instead a dihydronicotinic acid intermediate may be proposed which condenses with (6.64) leading to nicotine (6.71) (Scheme 6.15; H* corresponds to a C-6 tritium label) [50].

The combined results for nicotine suggest the pathway: ornithine (6.60) → putrescine (6.63) → (6.62) → (6.64) which condenses with a dihydronicotinic acid to give nicotine (6.71) (Scheme 6.15).

The biosynthesis of nicotinic acid in animals and some microorganisms is well established to be by degradation of tryptophan, whereas in plants nicotinic acid has its origins in aspartic acid and glycerol (glyceraldehyde) via quinolinic acid (6.72) (Scheme 6.16).

HO$_2$C   HOCH$_2$ OH   HO$_2$C   HO$_2$C

HO$_2$C   NH$_2$ R   HO$_2$C   N   N

Aspartic   Glycerol, R = CH$_2$OH   (6.72)   Nicotinic acid
acid   Glyceraldehyde, R = CHO   Quinolinic acid

Scheme 6.16

Such are the origins of the pyridine ring in nicotine (6.71) [and anabasine (6.20), Section 6.2.1] as well as several other pyridine alkaloids [51].

The observed occurrence of hygrine (6.2) and tropane alkaloids, e.g. (6.67), in plants of the same species together with a consideration of their structures and the biosynthesis of nicotine (6.71) and piperidine alkaloids already discussed, indicates the sequence of biosynthesis for e.g. hyoscyamine (6.67), shown in Scheme 6.13. This is supported by the observed incorporations of hygrine (6.2) and tropine (6.66) into hyoscyamine (6.67). Hygrine is also a precursor for cuscohygrine (6.68). Interestingly, and correctly, [N-methyl, 2'-^{14}C$_2$]hygrine [as (6.2)] gave (6.68) where the *specific* radioactivity in the N-methyl groups of the alkaloid was one half of that required to maintain the N-methyl: C-2' ratio of radioactivity from the hygrine [52]. Thus the second pyrrolidine ring of cuscohygrine arises not by degradation of hygrine but by condensation of the side-chain methyl group of hygrine with a further molecule of (6.64).

Tropine (6.66) is a precursor for the more extensively oxygenated alkaloids, scopolamine (6.73) and meteloidine (6.75), presumably by way of (6.74) [53, 54]. The two oxygenation sequences involve loss of the C-6 and C-7 β-protons from (6.66) [55].

(6.73) Scopolamine   (6.74)   (6.75) Meteloidine

Scheme 6.17

The tropane alkaloids commonly occur as esters of tropic acid [as (6.67)] and tiglic acid [as (6.75)]. The former acid arises preferentially from phenylalanine possibly via cinnamic acid and the entire carbon skeleton is involved. The results of ^{14}C-labelling studies show that, in the rearrangement which occurs during biosynthesis, it is the carboxy group which migrates (see Scheme 6.18). Proof of an

Phenylalanine   (6.76) Tropic acid

Scheme 6.18

intramolecular shift for this group was obtained by showing that [1,3-^{13}C$_2$]phenylalanine (majority of molecules doubly labelled) afforded *doubly* labelled hyoscyamine (6.67) and scopolamine (6.73), with labels confined to the expected sites. (Intermolecular migration would have led to two singly labelled species due to dilution with unlabelled materials in the plant [56, 57].) It is interesting to note a similar biosynthesis for a related system in the microbial metabolite tenellin (Section 7.2), which argues for a rearrangement characteristic of phenylalanine metabolism rather than of a particular secondary metabolite.

The biosynthesis of the tigloyl [as (6.75)] residues of, e.g., meteloidine (6.75), has been found to be similar to that leading to tiglic acid in animals. It derives from the amino acid L-isoleucine [58–60].

Various carboxylic acids are found as the necic acid parts of the pyrrolizidine alkaloids, e.g. senecionine (6.77), monocrotaline (6.78) and heliosupine (6.79). Available evidence [61, 62] points to the derivation of these acids from the branched-chain amino acids isoleucine and valine (see dotted lines). [In the case of monocrotaline C-4, C-5, and C-8 apparently derive from propionic acid. Carbon atoms 5 and 6 of the echimidinic acid fragment in (6.79) apparently derive from acetate.] The basic fragment in these alkaloids, retronecine (6.80), is formed [63] from two molecules of

Isoleucine

(6.77) Senecionine
(2 x Isoleucine)

(6.78) Monocrotaline
(1 x Isoleucine)

Angelic acid
(1xIsoleucine)

Echimidinic acid
(1 x Valine)

Valine

(6.79) Heliosupine

ornithine via putrescine (distinction between C-2 and C-5 of the amino acid is lost) (see Scheme 6.19).

Putrescine

Scheme 6.19

(6.80)

The phenanthroindolizidine alkaloids, e.g. tylophorine (6.81), are formed in *Tylophora asthmatica* from a molecule each of tyrosine and phenylalanine (see Scheme 6.20), with ornithine apparently the

Phenylalanine

Tyrosine

(6.81) Tylophorine

Scheme 6.20

source of ring E. The intact incorporation of the phenacylpyr-rolidines (6.84), (6.85) and (6.86) provided important information on the steps of biosynthesis [64]. [It is because of the involvement of these compounds in biosynthesis and the close structural similarity to, *inter alia*, hygrine (6.2), that discussion of the biosynthesis of these alkaloids appears here.]

In addition, the keto acids (6.82) and (6.83) were intact precursors [a common sequence, *in vivo*, is phenylalanine → cinnamic acid → (6.82)]. The late stages of biosynthesis were suggested by the structure (6.88) for the naturally occurring base, septicine, i.e. that linkage between the aromatic rings of the amino acid fragments to give the phenanthrene system of (6.81), would occur by oxidative phenol coupling (Section 1.3.1), and at a late stage of biosynthesis. With this in mind examination of the structures (6.81), (6.91) and (6.92) of the *T. asthmatica* alkaloids indicated that (6.89) could be a key intermediate for the formation of all three alkaloids [65].

Samples of (6.87), (6.89) and (6.93), double labelled as shown (* = ^{3}H, ● = ^{14}C), were found to be incorporated into (6.81), (6.91) and (6.92) at a similar level in each alkaloid, indicating a close biosynthetic relationship between the alkaloids. The changes in isotope ratio were consistent with necessary loss of tritium from sites in (6.87) and (6.93) which became hydroxylated in the course of

Scheme 6.21

biosynthesis and from C-6′ in (*6.89*) during phenol coupling. It follows from this that (*6.87*), (*6.89*) and (*6.93*) are intact precursors* for (*6.81*), (*6.91*) and (*6.92*), but the much lower incorporation observed for (*6.93*) compared with the other two compounds indicated that it was utilized along a minor pathway. The major route to the alkaloids must be as shown (Scheme 6.21). The indolizidine (*6.89*) can only give (*6.81*), (*6.91*) and (*6.92*) via the dienone (*6.90*), alternative courses of rearrangement (path b, Scheme 6.21), and reduction and rearrangement (path a) affording the three alkaloids after further minor modification. In the rearrangement of (*6.90*) (and the dienol derived from it), the unique opportunity, in alkaloid biosynthesis, of styryl (as against aryl, see Section 6.3) migration must be taken in affording (*6.91*) and (*6.92*), and it may well be taken in the formation of (*6.81*).

6.3 Isoquinoline and related alkaloids

6.3.1 *Phenethylamines and simple isoquinolines*
The simplest of the phenethylamine alkaloids are *N*-methyltyramine (*6.96*) and hordenine (*6.97*), which are found in barley roots. Their genesis is an appropriately simple one from the aromatic amino acid tyrosine (*6.94*) via tyramine (*6.95*), with methionine serving as the source for the *N*-methyl groups [66, 67]. The biosynthesis of mescaline (*6.107*), the hallucinogen from the peyote cactus, has similar beginnings in tyrosine and tyramine. Extensive experimentation, including that with an *O*-methyltransferase from peyote, has allowed mapping of the biosynthetic pathways in detail (see Scheme 6.22) [68, 69]. A key stage is reached with the formation of (*6.102*). Methylation of the hydroxy-group at C-3 leads to mescaline (*6.107*), whereas methylation of the alternative at C-4 leads to the isoquinoline alkaloids anhalonidine (*6.110*) and anhalamine (*6.109*).

All except one and two carbon atoms in the skeletons of, respectively, (*6.109*) and (*6.110*), are accounted for by phenethylamine (*6.101*). The origins of these almost trivial C_1/C_2 units proved quite elusive until a suggestion of some thirty years' standing, namely that (*6.104*) and (*6.105*) could be precursors for (*6.110*) and (*6.109*), respectively, was examined with positive results. The amine (*6.101*) and pyruvic acid, both precursors for anhalonidine (*6.110*), reacted together readily *in vitro* to give (*6.104*) (see Scheme 6.23), which was a specific precursor *in vivo* for anhalonidine (*6.110*). It was shown to be a constituent of peyote and was decarboxylated by fresh peyote slices to the imine (*6.106*) which was then established as a further biosynthetic intermediate [70]. A similar route accounts for the formation of

*For discussion of the use of doubly-labelled precursors to test for intact incorporation see Sections 2.2.1 and 6.4.2.

Scheme 6.22

anhalamine (*6.109*), via (*6.105*) which is derived from glyoxylic acid rather than pyruvic acid [70]. Salsoline (*6.108*) was subsequently shown to be derived along a related pathway and the key benzyliso-quinoline alkaloid, norlaudanosoline (*6.123*), forms similarly by way of (*6.121*) (Scheme 6.24). A related pathway may be adduced for the unusual alkaloid lophocerine (*6.115*) from leucine, which is a proven precursor. A separate derivation for the C_5 unit (C-1 plus isobutyl group) in this alkaloid has been deduced [71, 72] to be mevalonate by way of (*6.111*), (*6.112*) and (*6.113*), all of which serve as lophocerine precursors. Isoquinoline formation along this route involves perforce an aldehyde in contrast to the α-carbonyl acids utilized for the biosynthesis of the other alkaloids discussed above. The formation of cryptostyline-I (*6.116*) also involves an aldehyde intermediate along an otherwise orthodox pathway from tyrosine [73]. In

(*6.117*) Macromerine

(*6.118*) Ephedrine

(*6.116*) Cryptostyline-I

sum it appears that amino acids of type (*6.104*) will be seen to have increasing, if not quite exclusive, importance as intermediates in the biosynthesis of a wide variety of alkaloids with a structural unit of type (*6.119*) (Scheme 6.23) (cf. Scheme 6.21). Biosynthesis involving the corresponding aldehyde will be strictly similar.

Scheme 6.23

(*6.119*)

† Some naturally occurring phenethylamines, e.g. macromerine (*6.117*), bear a hydroxy group in the β-position of the side-chain. Their origins are, however, unexceptionally in tyrosine. It appears that the distinguishing β-hydroxylation step may be an early one [74, 75]. Ephedrine (*6.118*) has a *C*-methyl group in its side-chain in addition to the β-hydroxy-group of bases like macromerine. Curiously, in spite of the structural kinship of (*6.118*) to bases like (*6.117*), the genesis of ephedrine (*6.118*) is quite different. Phenylalanine was incorporated (via cinnamic acid) but only as a C_6–C_1 unit. Benzoic acid and benzaldehyde were incorporated at a higher level and it seems possible that normal derivation of the C_6–C_1 unit in ephedrine (*6.118*) is directly from shikimic acid rather than via its metabolite phenylalanine [76] (Section 5.1). Methionine serves as the source of the *N*-methyl group of ephedrine, but the origin of the remaining C_2N group is obscure, except that aspartate or close relative may be involved.

The 1-benzyltetrahydroisoquinoline skeleton is one of pre-eminence in the elaboration of plant alkaloids. Only the terpenoid indole skeleton (Section 6.6.2) appears in more diversely modified form. Among the benzylisoquinolines, reticuline (*6.127*) is of outstanding importance as a substrate for modification. Formation of the

(6.123) Norlaudanosoline   (6.122)
Scheme 6.24

benzylisoquinoline skeleton follows the pathway shown in Scheme 6.24, from two molecules of tyrosine [77–80].

One of the simplest benzylisoquinolines is papaverine (6.124) which is formed from norlaudanosoline (6.123) [81–83]. The most complex are the bisbenzylisoquinolines, e.g. epistephanine (6.125), and so far it is established that coclaurine (6.126) is a key precursor for several of these alkaloids [84–86]. Coclaurine itself has a genesis similar to that outlined in Scheme 6.24 [87].

(6.124) Papaverine   (6.125)   (6.126) Coclaurine

6.3.2 Aporphines

All that is required for the transformation of the benzylisoquinoline skeleton [as (6.123)] into that of the aporphines, e.g. bulbocapnine (6.129), is a single new bond. Clearly phenol oxidative coupling (N.B. see Section 1.3.1) is involved here, but there are several possible routes to a particular alkaloid. Interestingly examples of most of these possibilities have been found for the biosynthesis of one or more of the aporphine alkaloids, and in one case, that of boldine (6.131), biosynthesis takes a different course in two different plants. Methylation pattern in the alkaloid produced does not provide a reliable guide to the course of biosynthesis, as witness that of (6.131) in Scheme 6.25 [88]. The methylation pattern suggests a different pathway (see Scheme 6.27), which is followed in another plant.

The simplest biosynthetic sequence is found in bulbocapnine (6.129). Oxidative coupling occurs here between the sites *ortho* to the

(6.127) Reticuline   (6.128)   (6.129) Bulbocapnine

(6.130) Isoboldine   (6.131) Boldine

Scheme 6.25

two hydroxy groups in reticuline (6.127) to give (6.128) which with minor modification affords (6.129) [89] (for the mechanism of methylene-dioxy-group formation see Section 6.4.1, Scheme 6.36). Reticuline (6.127) is a proved precursor for two other aporphines [90, 91].

The importance of O-methylation pattern in deciding the course of coupling is well illustrated by results of a study on the biosynthesis of thebaine (6.151) and isothebaine (6.135) which are both natural constituents of *Papaver orientale*. Whereas reticuline (6.127) is modified to give thebaine (6.151) (Section 6.3.4) orientaline (6.132), differing from reticuline in the location of one methyl group, has a quite different fate in isothebaine (6.135). In other cases a precursor, with the wrong methylation pattern, fails to yield alkaloid.

Because the benzylisoquinoline skeleton derives from tyrosine (6.94) which has a phenolic hydroxy-group at C-4', the aporphines should have hydroxy-groups at equivalent positions. Isothebaine (6.135) lacks such a group at one expected site, C-10. It follows that a hydroxy-group is lost from this site in the course of biosynthesis, plausibly via 'dienol-benzene' rearrangement in (6.134) (see Section 1.3.1). This suggests the route shown in Scheme 6.26, which experiments have shown is correct [92]. Orientaline (6.132), and the key

(6.132) Orientaline   (6.133)   (6.134)   (6.135) Isothebaine

Scheme 6.26

dienone (6.133) were shown to be precursors. The latter was also found as a natural constituent of *P. orientale*. One of the dienols obtained on chemical reduction of (6.133) was a much more efficient precursor for isothebaine (6.135) than the other indicating stereospecificity, and hence enzyme catalysis, in the dienol-benzene rearrangement.

The structures of the *Dicentra eximia* bases, glaucine (6.138), dicentrine (6.140) and, particularly, corydine (6.139) indicate a similar pattern of biosynthesis to that already discussed. Quite unexpectedly the biosynthetic route turned out to be different. Painstaking work established [93] that biosynthesis is from norprotosinomenine (6.136); the likely following steps are indicated in Scheme 6.27 (the point of *N*-methylation is unknown). Boldine (6.131) is a logical, and

(6.136) Norprotosinomenine   (6.137) R³ = H or Me   (6.138) Glaucine

(6.139) Corydine   (6.140) Dicentrine

Scheme 6.27

proven, intermediate in the sequence to (6.138) and (6.140). Interestingly in the plant *Litsea glutinosa* boldine is formed from reticuline (6.127) via isoboldine (6.130) (Scheme 6.25) [88] [the conversion of (6.130) into (6.131), as observed in other examples, largely involves methyl loss and remethylation rather than methyl transfer].

A key role for dienones, e.g. (6.133) and (6.137), in aporphine alkaloid biosynthesis is apparent. Their importance is emphasized by their natural occurrence. One such is crotonosine (6.141) formed

(6.141) Crotonosine

from coclaurine (*6.126*) [94] which is also involved in the formation of related alkaloids [95, 96].

6.3.3 *Erythrina alkaloids*

The unusual structures of the *Erythrina* alkaloids, e.g. erythraline (*6.144*), suggest an unusual biogenesis. Although the later steps of biosynthesis are unusual, the first key intermediate is surprisingly a benzylisoquinoline: *N*-norprotosinomenine (*6.136*) (*S*-isomer), which is involved along with a dienone [as (*6.137*) = (*6.142*)] in the biosynthesis of both erythraline and some aporphine alkaloids (see above).

The pathway [97, 98] must involve a symmetrical intermediate because [2-^{14}C]tyrosine [as (*6.94*)] gave β-erythroidine (*6.147*) with equal labelling of C-8 and C-10, and more importantly because *N*-[4'-*methoxy*-^{14}C]norprotosinomenine [as (*6.136*)] gave erythraline (*6.144*) with equal labelling of methoxy- and methylenedioxy-groups.

Other intermediates in erythraline biosynthesis were proved to be (*6.143*), (*S*)-erysodienone (*6.146*), and 2-epierythratine [as (*6.145*)], and all the results are consistent with the suggested pathway (Scheme 6.28). The lactonic erythroidines, e.g. (*6.147*), arise from

Norprotosinomenine (*6.136*)

(*6.142*)

(*6.143*)

(*6.144*) Erythraline

(*6.145*) Erythratine

(*6.146*) Erysodienone

C-2 epimer

Scheme 6.28

(*6.147*)

bases of the erythraline type, in a sequence which manifestly involves aromatic ring scission—a rare thing in the biosynthesis of plant bases (cf. betalains, Section 6.8).

6.3.4   Morphine and related alkaloids

The idea that the opium alkaloid morphine is a modified benzylisoquinoline provided the key to the structure (6.152) for the alkaloid;
twisting of the benzylisoquinoline skeleton into that shown for
reticuline (6.127) in (6.148) illustrates this relationship and suggests a
possible biogenesis. This was later proved correct in the course of a
study which is one of the classics of alkaloid biosynthesis. In the first
experiments ever to be carried out with complex plant-alkaloid precursors, [1-^{14}C]- and [3-^{14}C]-norlaudanosoline [as (6.123)] were fed
to opium poppies [99, 100]. They were found to label morphine
(6.152), codeine (6.153) and thebaine (6.151) specifically, thus estab-
ishing that these alkaloids are indeed benzylisoquinoline derivatives.
The key intermediate [101] proved to be reticuline (6.148). Both (R)
and (S)-isomers were utilized, the latter by way of (6.155) [101, 102]
which allowed its conversion into (R)-reticuline (6.148), the 'correct'
intermediate, with the same configuration as the three opium
alkaloids [as (6.151)].

(6.148) (R)-Reticuline   (6.149) Salutaridine   (6.150)   (6.151) Thebaine

(6.152) Morphine   (6.153) Codeine   (6.154)

Scheme 6.29

Ortho-para oxidative coupling of the diphenol, reticuline (6.148),
can be conceived of as giving the dienone (6.149) which could afford
thebaine (6.151) as shown [101]. This hypothesis is strongly supported by the observation that this dienone, (6.149), called
salutaridine, is a constituent of opium poppies, is formed from
radioactive tyrosine (6.94) and norlaudanosoline (6.123), and is a
highly efficient and specific precursor for the opium alkaloids. The
transformation of salutaridine (6.149) into thebaine (6.151) requires a
further ring-closure, which occurs chemically when the two epimeric
alcohols (6.150) are treated with acid. In contrast to the purely
chemical reaction, only one of the alcohols was efficiently converted
into thebaine in vivo, indicating that the reaction is enzyme mediated
(and therefore part of normal biosynthesis).

Experiments, particularly with $^{14}CO_2$ [103, 104], have established that in the biosynthesis of the opium alkaloids thebaine (6.151) is the first alkaloid to be formed and the following sequence is essentially one of demethylation (Scheme 6.29). It is interesting to note that the demethylation at C-6 which converts thebaine (6.151) into (6.154), does not involve loss of the oxygen atom as expected of normal enol ether hydrolysis; a possible mechanism is shown in Scheme 6.30 [105].

Scheme 6.30

6.3.5 Hasubanonine and protostephanine

†Hasubanonine (6.158) and protostephanine (6.157) have structures which in the light of the foregoing discussion appear to be benzyliso-quinoline in origin. It took, however, really extensive, careful experiments to establish this [106], because the benzylisoquinoline substrate for oxidative coupling, i.e. (6.156), needed to have *two* hydroxy groups on ring B. This is quite unprecedented. In all other known examples only one hydroxy group per ring has been found to be necessary. The deduced pathway is illustrated in Scheme 6.31.

(6.157) Protostephanine   (6.158) Hasubanonine
Scheme 6.31

6.3.6   Protoberberine and related alkaloids

Elaboration of the benzylisoquinoline skeleton in ways different from those already discussed involve the inclusion of an extra carbon atom (the 'berberine bridge') as seen in, e.g. berberine (6.161) (the extra atom is C-8). The question of how this occurs was answered simply in terms of an oxidative cyclization of the N-methyl group of a benzylisoquinoline precursor in a manner (Scheme 6.32) analogous

(6.159) (S) - Reticuline

(6.160)

(6.161) Berberine

Scheme 6.32

to the formation of a methylenedioxy-group (Section 6.4.1; Scheme 6.36) (both the 'berberine bridge' and methylene-dioxy-carbons derive ultimately from methionine). The benzylisoquinoline was established to be reticuline (6.159) [utilized via canadine (6.160)] with (S)-isomer preferred to (R). Label in the N-methyl group of (6.159) was built intact into C-8 of berberine, thus validating the hypothesis [107–109].

† The early suspicion that chelidonine (6.165) was a protoberberine [as (6.162)] variant has been confirmed [109–113]. The deduced route, which includes another alkaloid protopine (6.164) and begins with the ubiquitous precursor reticuline, is illustrated in Scheme 6.33. Tritium-labelling results establish that C-1 and C-9 of reticuline (6.159) are unaffected by transformation through scoulerine (6.162) to stylopine (6.163). The conversion of the N-methyl group of reticuline into the 'berberine bridge' (C-8) of stylopine (6.163), which necessarily involves loss of one hydrogen/tritium atom, was found to occur with very high retention of tritium label on this carbon atom, consistent with the expected operation of an isotope effect favouring loss of hydrogen rather than tritium. Subsequent transformation of stylopine (6.163) to chelidonine occurs with retention of tritium at C-5 and C-8, but loss of tritium from C-14 and the (pro-S)-hydrogen atoms from C-13 and C-6 (loss in each case of a proton from the α-face of the biosynthetic intermediates is notable).

† The phthalideisoquinoline alkaloids, e.g. hydrastine (6.166), also

(6.162) (S)-Scoulerine

(6.163) (S)-Stylopine

(6.164) Protopine

(6.165) Chelidonine

Scheme 6.33

derive from (S)-scoulerine (6.162). Entry of the C-13 oxygen atom occurs with removal of the *pro-S* proton (as in chelidonine biosynthesis), and the reaction thus proceeds with orthodox retention of configuration [110–112].

† Corydaline (6.167), ochotensimine (6.168) [114] and alpinigenine (6.170) are further protoberberine variants; the labelling of (6.167) and (6.168) by [3-¹⁴C]tyrosine [as (6.94); ●] and methionine (*; includes 'berberine-bridge' atom) is shown. Alpinigenine (6.170) is formed via the protopine relative (6.169) [115, 116].

6.3.7 Phenylethylisoquinoline alkaloids

Colchicine (6.175) is an alkaloid with a unique tropolone ring, and on the face of it appears to be quite unrelated to any other alkaloid.

(6.166) Hydrastine   (6.167) Corydaline   (6.168) Ochotensimine

(6.169)   (6.170) Alpinigenine

Phenylalanine, by way of cinnamic acid, serves in *Colchicum* species as the source of ring A plus carbon atoms 5, 6, and 7. The seven carbons of the tropolone ring arise from tyrosine which loses C-1 and C-2 from the side-chain; labels from [4'-^{14}C]- and [3-^{14}C]-labelled amino acid appear at C-9 and C-12, respectively [117]. It follows that the tropolone ring arises by expansion of the tyrosine benzene ring with inclusion of the benzylic carbon atom, but through what series of intermediates?

The answer came from the elucidation of the structure of androcymbine, an alkaloid isolated from a relative of *Colchicum*. The dienone structure (6.173) was assigned to androcymbine. Androcymbine could then be thought of as arising from the phenethyliso-

(6.171) (S) - Autumnaline

(6.172) R=Me
(6.173) R=H, Androcymbine

(6.174)

(6.175) Colchicine

Scheme 6.34

quinoline skeleton [as (6.171)] which was quite unknown at the time [118]. A similar biogenesis for colchicine followed. Plausibly the transformation of the androcymbine skeleton (6.173) to that of colchicine could occur by hydroxylation to give (6.174). Homoallylic ring expansion would lead to colchicine (Scheme 6.34).

The crucial test for the hypothesis lay in the examination of compounds of type (6.171) and (6.173) as colchicine precursors. In the event [119–121], O-methylandrocymbine (6.172) was a spectacularly good precursor for colchicine. The phenethylisoquinoline (6.171), called autumnaline, was also clearly implicated in biosynthesis; only the (S)-isomer of autumnaline, with the same absolute configuration as colchicine is involved, and oxidative coupling of this base occurs in a para-para sense rather than the alternative, ortho-para. Results of other experiments, together with those discussed here, led to the pathway illustrated in Scheme 6.34.

†   Autumnaline (6.176) is a precursor for homoaporphine alkaloids, e.g. floramultine (6.177), found in Kreysigia multiflora [122]. The homo-Erythrina alkaloid, schelhammeridine (6.178) [123], and cephalotaxine (6.179) [124] are apparently also modified phenethylisoquinolines.

(6.176)   (6.177) Floramultine   (6.178) Schelhammeridine

(6.179) Cephalotaxine

6.4   Amaryllidaceae and mesembrine alkaloids

The grouping of these two groups of alkaloids together can be justified on a certain structural resemblance and on a derivation from the same amino acids. But they are derived along apparently different pathways appropriate to the phylogenetically different plants which produce the two groups of alkaloids.

6.4.1   Amaryllidaceae alkaloids

Diverse though the structures of these alkaloids seem they may be classified into three main groups represented by (6.185), (6.187) and (6.190). The quite brilliant recognition that the three groups of alkaloids could arise simply by different modes of phenol oxidative coupling (Section 1.3.1) within a molecule of type (6.180) has been of central importance to biosynthetic studies in this area, studies which were to prove the correctness of the original idea.

Examination of (6.180) indicates an assembly from a C_6–C_1 and a C_6–C_2 unit (thickened bonds) which can be traced through into the alkaloids (6.185), (6.187) and (6.190). It was established for representative alkaloids by the results of feeding radioactive compounds, that the C_6–C_2 unit arises from tyrosine (a common source for such units) via tyramine and that the C_6–C_1 unit arises from phenylalanine (a common source of C_6–C_1 and C_6–C_3 units) by way of cinnamic acid, its 3,4-dihydroxy-derivative, and protocatechualdehyde (6.184) [125–128]. It is interesting to note that, as is often the case in plant alkaloid biosynthesis, hydroxylation of phenylalanine to give tyrosine

(6.180) Norbelladine   (6.181) O-Methylnorbelladine   (6.182) R=H, Norpluviine
(6.183) R=Me

(6.184)

(6.185) Lycorine

(6.186) Oxocrinine

(6.187) R=H, Haemanthamine
(6.188) R=OH

(6.189)

(6.190) R¹=H, R²=Me, Galanthamine
(6.191) R¹=Me, R²=H

Scheme 6.35

does not occur (as also colchicine, Section 6.3.7, but not capsaicin [129, 130] or annuloline [131]).

Further experimental results established norbelladine (*6.180*) and some of its methylated derivatives (clearly not others) as key biosynthetic intermediates in the biosynthesis of, e.g., lycorine (*6.185*), haemanthamine (*6.187*) and galanthamine (*6.190*) [125–128, 132, 133]. As elsewhere (see Section 6.3) hydroxy-groups *ortho* and/or *para* to sites of new bond formation between aromatic rings are essential for biosynthesis to proceed, a telling set of examples in support of the phenol-oxidative coupling hypothesis. Of further interest is the reported isolation of an enzyme, from a plant of the Amaryllidaceae, which, when incubated with norbelladine and S-adenosylmethionine (source of methyl groups), yielded almost entirely the O-methylnorbelladine, (*6.181*), that is involved in alkaloid biosynthesis [134].

In the course of studies on the incorporation of O-[*methyl*-^{14}C]methylnorbelladine [as (*6.181*)] into haemanthamine (*6.187*) it was demonstrated [128], for the first time, that a methylene-dioxy-group [as in (*6.187*)] arises by oxidative ring closure of an *o*-methoxyphenol [as in (*6.181*)]. Subsequent results on the biosynthesis of other alkaloids have confirmed the generality of this observation. The mechanism may be one involving radicals or cationic species (Scheme 6.36). A related oxidative cyclization is found in the conversion of an isoquinoline into a protoberberine (Section 6.3.6) where an N-methyl group closes on to an aromatic ring.

Scheme 6.36

The deduced pathway to galanthamine (*6.190*) which involves *ortho-para* oxidative coupling is illustrated in Scheme 6.35; chlidanthine (*6.191*) is formed from galanthamine (*6.190*) [135]. Similar coupling but in the opposite sense (*para-ortho*) leads to norpluviine (*6.182*) and by allylic hydroxylation on to lycorine (*6.185*) [125]; further oxidation, this time of galanthine (*6.192*), gives narcissidine (*6.193*) [136]. The retention of two out of four tritium atoms in the formation of norpluviine (*6.182*) from O-methylnorbelladine [labelled

(6.192) (6.193)

as shown in (6.194)] requires a complex pathway (b, Scheme 6.37) rather than a simpler one (path a) which would result in the retention of three tritium atoms [132].

Scheme 6.37

The hydroxylation of (6.182) to give lycorine (6.185) would be expected to proceed with retention of configuration, the orthodox result (see Section 1.2.3). It has been found, however, that although this is true for biosynthesis in one plant, the opposite is true in another plant [137, 138].

The third group of alkaloids which arise from norbelladine (6.180), this time by *para-para* phenol oxidative coupling, is exemplified by haemanthamine (6.187), and biosynthesis is proved to be by way of compounds of type (6.186). Haemanthamine (6.187) shows an extra hydroxy-group at C-11, which has been shown to arise by hydroxylation with normal retention of configuration [139, 140].

Haemanthamine (6.187) is a precursor for haemanthidine (6.188). The conversion of protocatechualdehyde (6.184) through the sequence (6.184) → (6.181) → (6.187) → haemanthidine (6.188) has been shown by the results of tritium labelling to involve stereospecific hydrogen addition to, and removal from, what begins as the aldehyde carbonyl, the hydrogen added being later removed [141]. A similar sequence has been found for the conversion of protocatechualdehyde (6.184) through (6.181) and (6.183) into lycorenine (6.196); the proton added and removed is the (7-*pro-R*) one in (6.183) [142].

† The structure (6.200) of narciclasine is such that it can *a priori* arise along a route involving intermediates of the norpluviine (6.182) or oxocrinine (6.186) types. Tracer experiments have shown that the latter route is utilized and involves *inter alia* oxocrinine (6.186) and vittatine (6.197). Loss of the two-carbon bridge in the conversion of (6.197) into (6.200) could plausibly occur as shown on 11-hydroxyvittatine (6.198). This is supported by the finding that

(6.196) Lycorenine

(6.197)

(6.198)

(6.199) Ismine

(6.200) Narciclasine

(6.198) is an efficient precursor for narciclasine (6.200) [143, 144] (cf. colchicine biosynthesis, Section 6.3.7, for a related fragmentation).

† More extensive skeletal degradation than that seen in narciclasine biosynthesis is apparent in the genesis of ismine (6.199). Results of tracer experiments have shown [145] that it too arises from oxoc-rinine (6.186), with loss of C-12 (so it does not become the N-methyl group of ismine) and the (6-pro-R)-hydrogen atom. Interestingly this is a proton with the same stereochemistry as those lost in haeman-thidine (6.188) and lycorenine (6.196) biosynthesis (see above).

† Some evidence [146, 147] exists that alkaloids of the manthine (6.201) type are formed from those of the haemanthamine (6.187) kind.

(6.201)

6.4.2 Mesembrine alkaloids

The group of alkaloids exemplified by mesembrine (6.202), shows a structural kinship with Amaryllidaceae alkaloids of the haeman-thamine (6.187) type. However, the only aspect of biosynthesis com-mon to these two groups of alkaloids is their origin in phenylalanine and tyrosine; results, crucially with doubly labelled precursors, showed that various norbelladine (6.180) derivatives were only incorporated after fragmentation [148].

The octahydroindole moiety in these alkaloids derives from tyrosine via tyramine, and N-methyltyramine [149]. Phenylalanine is the source of the unusual, if not unique, mesembrine C_6 unit. As with other metabolites phenylalanine is utilized by way of cinnamic acid and, in this case, mono- and di-hydroxy-derivatives may be involved too. Late-stage aromatic hydroxylation is also possible, for

(6.202) Mesembrine

Phenylalanine

N-Methyltyramine

↑

Tyrosine

Scheme 6.38

skeletenone *(6.203)* is an efficient precursor for mesembrenol *(6.205)* [150] and appears to be on the major pathway.

(6.203)   *(6.204)*   *(6.205)* Mesembrenol

The steps which lie immediately beyond hydroxy-cinnamic acids and *N*-methyltyramine remain a mystery, but possible intermediates are in part circumscribed by the results of experiments with tritiated precursors. Thus tritium at C-2' and C-6' of phenylalanine is retained on formation of mesembrine *(6.202)* [148]. Formation of intermediates [as *(6.186)*] would require loss of one tritium atom, so further independent evidence for disparate pathways to these two groups of alkaloids is obtained. Moreover, the results indicate that bond formation between the phenylalanine- and tyrosine-derived units must occur at the carbon atom corresponding to C-1' of phenylalanine. This leads logically to a dienone of type *(6.204)*, which can undergo fragmentation and aromatization as indicated without tritium loss. Cyclization of nitrogen on to C-7a [see *(6.205)*] must occur at some point. Half of the tritium from C-3' and C-5' of labelled tyrosine and *N*-methyltyramine was lost in mesembrenol *(6.205)* formation, residual tritium appearing at C-5 and C-7α (equal distribution of label between these sites indicates that tritium loss must occur whilst they are equivalent, i.e. before dienone formation). The results are consistent with the pathway shown, which involves internal conjugate addition of nitrogen to the enone followed by stereospecific β-protonation of the resulting enolate at C-7 [149].

6.5 Quinoline and related alkaloids

† A number of diverse alkaloids have a common anthranilic acid unit. This amino acid is an intermediate in tryptophan biosynthesis. The known pathways to some of the alkaloids, damascenine (*6.206*) [151], echinorine (*6.207*) [152], the benzoxazinone (*6.208*) [153], and graveoline (*6.210*) [154], are illustrated in Scheme 6.39. Further anthranilic acid derivatives are arborine (*6.211*) [155, 156], rutaecarpine

Scheme 6.39

(*6.212*) and evodiamine (*6.213*) (also derived from tryptophan) [157] and acridone alkaloids, e.g. melicopicine (*6.214*) [158, 159].

† Peganine (≡ vasicine) (*6.215*) is interesting because its biosynthesis appears to be along quite different pathways in two plants from different families (Scheme 6.40) [160–162]. This is so far a unique observation in plant alkaloid biosynthesis.

Scheme 6.40

† The furoquinoline alkaloids, e.g. platydesmine (6.220) and dictamnine (6.221), are derived from anthranilic acid, acetate (C_2 unit), and mevalonate (C_5 unit) [see dotted lines in (6.216) and (6.220)] along the pathway [163] shown in Scheme 6.41; prenylation of the

(6.216) R = H
(6.217) R = Me

(6.218) R = H
(6.219) R = Me

Mevalonic acid

(6.220) Platydesmine   (6.221) Dictamnine   (6.222) Skimmianine

Scheme 6.41

quinoline skeleton may occur as well with a methoxy-group at C-4 as with a hydroxy-group, because both (6.216) and (6.217), and (6.218) and (6.219) are efficient precursors [(6.219) being proven to be incorporated without loss of its methyl group], but methylation of the C-2 oxygen function prevents utilization in biosynthesis.

† The conversion of platydesmine (6.220) into dictamnine (6.221) involves loss of the isopropyl group from C-2. A mechanism involving stereospecific hydroxylation at C-3 [of (6.220)], followed by fragmentation (Scheme 6.42), was suggested by the observation that

Platydesmine
(6.220)

Dictamnine
(6.221)

(6.223)

Scheme 6.42

(6.219) was incorporated into skimmianine (6.222) with loss of half of a tritium label sited at C-1′ [of (6.219)]. An alternative mechanism could be one initiated by hydride abstraction from (6.220) instead of hydroxyl loss from (6.223).

† Further results have been obtained with cell suspension cultures of *Ruta graveolens*, which produces furoquinoline alkaloids and edulinine (6.224). In particular, (6.216) was deduced [164] to be at the branch point for the biosynthesis of the two alkaloid types, with *N*-methylation of (6.216) causing diversion to edulinine biosynthesis. The pathway to (6.224) also involves the *N*-methyl derivative of (6.219).

(6.224) Edulinine

6.6   Indole alkaloids

6.6.1   Simple indole derivatives

The simple base gramine (6.227) is known to derive from tryptophan (6.225), in three plants from different families. C-2 is lost but
apparently not the side-chain nitrogen [165].

(6.225) R = CO$_2$H, Tryptophan   (6.227) Gramine
(6.226) R = H, Tryptamine

(6.228) R = H
(6.229) R = PO$_3^{2-}$, Psilocybin

(6.230) R = H
(6.231) R = OMe

† Psilocybin (6.229) derives along the pathway: tryptophan
(6.225) → tryptamine (6.226) → N-methyltryptamine → N,N-dimethyl-
tryptamine → psilocin (6.228) = psilocybin (6.229) [166]. The biosynthesis of (6.230) and (6.231) is more complex. Almost all the possible
pathways from tryptophan (6.225) (made up of alternative sequences
of decarboxylation, hydroxylation, and O- and N-methylation)
appear to operate [167]. Such results are a caution against the simplistic
belief in a single biosynthetic pathway to secondary metabolites.

† The β-carboline alkaloids, e.g. harman (6.232) [168], also derive
from tryptophan as do the dimeric bases, calycanthine (6.234) and
folicanthine (6.233) [169]. These latter alkaloids are both plausibly
methyltryptamine dimers.

(6.232) Harman   (6.233) Folicanthine   (6.234) Calycanthine

6.6.2   Terpenoid indole and related alkaloids

The terpenoid indole skeleton is the most widely found amongst the
plant alkaloids, the number of known examples exceeding one
thousand. As seen in e.g. ajmalicine (6.243) these alkaloids are constituted from a tryptamine unit (proved to derive from tryptophan
and tryptamine [170]) and a C$_9$ or C$_{10}$ unit which, after much
experimentation, was proved to be terpenoid in origin. [Examination
of (6.243) shows this is not immediately obvious.]

Significant variation in the alkaloidal tryptamine fragment is associated with loss of one or both side-chain carbon atoms [see (6.272)] or transformation of the aromatic nucleus into that of a quinoline [see (6.275)]. By far the greatest variation is associated with the terpenoid fragment.

The most important, indeed crucial, idea put forward on the biosynthesis of these alkaloids was that they are formed by fragmentation of a cyclopentane monoterpene [as (6.237)]. The pathway outlined in Scheme 6.43 indicates how the major skeletal types represented by ajmalicine (6.243) and akuammicine (6.242), catharanthine (6.239), and vindoline (6.244) may be formed; where one of

(6.235) (R)-Mevalonic acid   (6.236) Geraniol   (6.237)   (6.238)

(6.239) Catharanthine   (6.240)   (6.241)

(6.242) Akuammicine   (6.243) Ajmalicine

Scheme 6.43   (6.244) Vindoline

these atoms is absent in derived alkaloids it appears always to be the one separated by dotted lines in (6.238), (6.240) and (6.241) [171, 172].

The appropriate incorporations of mevalonic acid (6.235) [as elsewhere in biosynthesis it is the (3-R)-isomer which is utilized], and geraniol (6.236) and nerol (6.245) prove the essential correctness of the hypothesis; the hydroxy-derivatives (6.246) and (6.247) were also utilized. Ensuing crucial experiments lay with identification of the cyclopentane monoterpene loganin (6.249) as a key intermediate in biosynthesis. Not only did (6.249) prove to be a specific alkaloid precursor, but its presence and biosynthesis from geraniol in *Catharanthus roseus*, a plant used for most of the experiments, could be demonstrated [173, 174].

Mevalonic acid → Geraniol *(6.236)*
(6.235)

(6.245) Nerol

(6.246)

(6.247)

MeO₂C *(6.248)*
—O-Glucose

(6.249) Loganin
MeO₂C
—O-Glucose

(6.250)

CHO
—O-Glucose
MeO₂C
(6.251) Secologanin

Scheme 6.44

Deoxyloganin (*6.248*) is sited as an intermediate before loganin (*6.249*) and cyclization of a geraniol precursor leading to it has been suggested to be as shown in Scheme 6.45; C-9 and C-10 become equivalent in this pathway as both are depicted as aldehydes, and this allows for the observation that label passing through (*6.236*) from mevalonate becomes equally divided between C-9 and C-10 of loganin (*6.249*) [175].

CHO   CHO   CHO
Me → Me ⇌ Me → Loganin
CHO CHO OH *(6.249)*

Scheme 6.45

Conversion of loganin (*6.249*) into alkaloids must involve cleavage of the cyclopentane ring [cf. (*6.249*) → (*6.251*) in Scheme 6.44], which may be rationalized in terms of the mechanism shown in (*6.250*) to give secologanin (*6.251*). This is corroborated by the firm identification of this terpene, (*6.251*), as a biosynthetic intermediate [176]. Consideration of the next step in biosynthesis leads to vincoside (*6.252*) and strictosidine (*6.253*) the epimeric products of chemical condensation between tryptamine (*6.226*) and secologanin (*6.251*). Recent results [177, 178] have shown that strictosidine (*6.253*) with 3α-stereochemistry is the precursor for alkaloids like ajmalicine (*6.243*) with 3α-stereochemistry [and also vindoline (*6.244*) and catharanthine (*6.239*)] and alkaloids similar to (*6.243*) but with 3β-stereochemistry. For the former group tritium at C-3 in (*6.253*) is retained, for those with 3β-stereochemistry it is lost (cf. ipecac alkaloids, Section 6.7 for slightly different results).

The most recent results [179, 180] have been obtained chiefly using enzyme preparations from plant tissue cultures, and they are most impressive allowing clear definition of the early stages of biosynthesis. Thus only strictosidine (*6.253*) is the product of *enzymic* condensation between tryptamine and secologanin (*6.251*). It accumulates in the presence of a β-glucosidase inhibitor [which blocks removal of the glucose in (*6.253*) and thus prevents further biosynthesis]. In the absence of inhibitor biosynthesis can proceed normally and the alkaloids, ajmalicine (*6.243*), its C-19 epimer, (*6.259*), and tetrahydroalstonine (*6.260*) are formed. The enzyme preparation required reduced pyridine nucleotide (**NADPH** or **NADH**) and, in the absence of coenzyme, cathenamine (*6.257*) accumulated. It was subsequently identified as an alkaloid in a plant, and was moreover enzymically converted into (*6.243*), (*6.259*) and (*6.260*) in the presence of NADPH. It is thus clearly an intermediate in biosynthesis as is logically (*6.254*). Evidence [181] in support was obtained by trapping (*6.254*) in reduced form from a *C. roseus* enzyme preparation incubated with strictosidine and potassium borohydride.

The *Corynanthé* alkaloids represented by ajmalicine (*6.243*) and tetrahydroalstonine (*6.260*) are the simplest variations of the stric-

Scheme 6.46

tosidine skeleton. Formation of an extra carbocyclic ring [as shown in (6.261)] affords yohimbine (6.262).

Simple rearrangement of the *Corynanthé* skeleton [as (6.243)] affords the *Strychnos* type, exemplified by akuammicine (6.242), and strychnine (6.263). Like (6.242), strychnine has been found to have the expected origins in tryptophan and in mevalonate via geraniol; the extra C_2 unit (C-22 and C-23) arises from acetate. Late intermediates have been identified and the pathway deduced is shown in Scheme 6.47 [182].

	19-H	20-H
(6.259)	α	β
(6.260)	β	α

(6.261)

(6.262) Yohimbine

Corynanthé skeleton →

(6.263) Strychnine

Scheme 6.47

It is, *a priori*, a reasonable hypothesis that alkaloids like catharanthine (6.239) (*Iboga* type) and vindoline (6.244) (*Aspidosperma* type) are formed by rearrangement of the *Corynanthé* skeleton [as (6.243)]. This is supported first by the observation that *Corynanthé* bases appear in *C. roseus* seedlings before *Iboga* and *Aspidosperma* alkaloids; second by the observation that the *Corynanthé* base, geissoschizine (6.258) is an intact precursor for representatives of the *Aspidosperma* and *Iboga* groups, and also those with the *Strychnos* skeleton [183, 184]. [Experiments [185] with an enzyme preparation of *C. roseus* tissue cultures indicate that geissoschizine is a shunt from the main biosynthetic pathway (in tissue cultures at least) (see Scheme 6.46). The deduced relationship between the alkaloid groups still stands, however.]

Results of orthodox feeding experiments, and those where the sequence of alkaloid formation is obtained by noting the appearance of precursor label in individual alkaloids in relation to time, have led to the conclusion that preakuammicine (6.264), stemmadenine (6.265) and tabersonine (6.266) are further important intermediates in the biosynthesis of both *Aspidosperma* [as (6.244)] and *Iboga* [as (6.239)] alkaloid types [186].

The formation of tabersonine (6.266) may be rationalized in terms of the sequence shown in Scheme 6.48, central to which is the enamine (6.267) formed by fragmentation of stemmadenine (6.265). *Iboga* alkaloids, e.g. catharanthine (6.239), are reasonably derivable from the enamine (6.267) also. If this is correct then the observed incorporation of labelled tabersonine (6.266) into catharanthine (6.239) indicates that (6.267) → (6.266) is reversible.

Scheme 6.48

The validity of (6.267) as a biosynthetic intermediate is supported by the isolation of simple secodine (6.268) derivatives from plants and by the specific incorporation of labelled secodine (6.268) into vindoline (6.244); the tritium loss from (6.268) labelled in the dihydropyridine ring on transformation into vindoline (6.244) is consistent with involvement of secodine (6.268) via a more highly oxidized intermediate [as (6.267)] [187].

Investigation of the biosynthesis of the bisindole alkaloid, vinblastine (6.270), has shown that it does, as expected, arise from catharanthine (6.239) and vindoline (6.244) probably by the mechanism shown in (6.269) [188, 189].

Vincamine (6.271), with a skeleton different from that discussed so far, is derived via tabersonine (6.266) [190]. In another different alkaloid, appicaricine (6.272), loss of one of the tryptamine side-chain carbons is apparent, and this appears to happen at a stage beyond stemmadenine (6.265) [191].

The *Cinchona* alkaloid, quinine (6.276), does not immediately seem

Secodine *(6.268)*

(6.269)

(6.270) Vinblastine

(6.271) Vincamine

(6.272) Apparicine

(6.273) Camptothecin

to be related to the alkaloids under discussion, but at quite an early date such a relationship was apparent since, e.g., cinchonamine *(6.274)* was also identified as a *Cinchona* base. It seemed 'likely, moreover, that alkaloids of type *(6.274)* would turn out to be intermediates in the formation of alkaloids like quinine *(6.276)*. This has been proved to be correct. The pathway, which the experimental results indicate [192], is illustrated in Scheme 6.49. Another

(6.274)

Strictosidine *(6.253)*

Scheme 6.49

(6.275) R=H, Cinchonidine
(6.276) R=OMe, Quinine

quinoline alkaloid is camptothecin *(6.273)*. It is formed by diversion at the strictosidine *(6.253)* stage, by lactam formation [reaction of N_b with the ester function of *(6.253)* rather than the aldehyde function] [193, 194].

6.7 Ipecac alkaloids [178, 195, 196]

† Part of the structure of the ipecac alkaloids, e.g. emetine *(6.281)* and cephaeline *(6.280)* [heavy bonding in *(6.280)*] is closely similar to the terpenoid fragment of the alkaloids just discussed (Section 6.6.2); the remaining atoms are accounted for by two phenethylamine units. Investigations which have paralleled those of the terpenoid indole alkaloids have established the origins of these alkaloids (see Scheme 6.50). Desacetylisoipecoside *(6.277)* is the key intermediate for *(6.280)*

Secologanin

(6.277) R = H
(6.278) R = H, C-5 epimer
(6.279) R = Ac, C-5 epimer

(6.280) R = H, Cephaeline
(6.281) R = Me, Emetine

Scheme 6.50

and *(6.281)*. It is the analogue of strictosidine *(6.253)* in the other group of alkaloids. Ipecoside *(6.279)* and alangiside *(6.282)* with

(6.282)

opposite stereochemistry at C-5 to *(6.277)* are derived not from *(6.277)* but from *(6.278)*, i.e. the precursor with the same stereochemistry unlike the situation with terpenoid indole alkaloids where *(6.253)* is the precursor for both of the corresponding epimeric series.

6.8 Miscellaneous alkaloids

† The biosynthesis of steroidal and terpenoid alkaloids can be correlated with the appropriate steroid and terpenoid precursors (Chapter 4).

Histidine, R = CO₂H
Histamine, R = H

(6.283) Dolichotheline

Scheme 6.51

† Alkaloids with unusual origins are dolichotheline (*6.283*), see Scheme 6.51 [197, 198], and shihunine (*6.285*) which derives from (*6.284*) [199] an important precursor for 1,4-naphthoquinones (cf. Section 5.2).

(6.284)   *(6.285)* Shihunine

† The betalains, e.g. betanin (*6.287*) and indicaxanthin (*6.288*), are coloured bases found in plants of the Centrospermae order. They have a well-defined function, e.g. as the pigments of some flowers. The pathway deduced for their biosynthesis is shown in Scheme 6.52. Notable is the exceptional extra-diol cleavage of the dopa unit

Scheme 6.52   *(6.288)* Indicaxanthin

which goes to make up the betalamic acid moiety (*6.286*) in (*6.287*) and (*6.288*) [200, 201].

References

Further reading: Herbert, R. B. (1979), in *Comprehensive Organic Chemistry* (eds. D. H. R. Barton and W. D. Ollis), Pergamon, Oxford, vol. 5, pp. 1045–119. Herbert, R. B. (1980), in *Rodd's Chemistry of Carbon Compounds* (ed. S. Coffey), 2nd Edn, Elsevier, Amsterdam, vol. IVL, pp. 291–455. [2]. Spenser, I. D. (1968), in *Comprehensive Biochemistry* (eds. M. Florkin and E. H. Stotz), Elsevier, Amsterdam, vol. 20, pp. 231–413. Dalton, D. R. (1979), *The Alkaloids, The Fundamental Chemistry, A Biogenetic Approach*, Dekker, New York. *Chemistry of The Alkaloids* (1970), (ed. S. W. Pelletier), van Nostrand Reinhold, New York.

[1] *The Alkaloids* (ed. R. H. F. Manske), Academic Press, New York, now approx. sixteen volumes.

[2] *The Alkaloids*, (*Specialist Periodical Reports*) [ed. J. E. Saxton (vols. 1–5), ed. M. F. Grundon (vols. 6–10)], The Chemical Society, London.

[3] Robinson, R. (1955), *The Structural Relations of Natural Products*, Oxford University Press, Oxford.

[4] Leete, E. and Slattery, S. A. (1976), *J. Amer. Chem. Soc.*, **98**, 6326–30.

[5] Leete, E. (1977), *Phytochemistry*, **16**, 1705–9.

[6] Leete, E. and Olson, J. O. (1972), *J. Amer. Chem. Soc.*, **94**, 5472–7.

[7] Roberts, M. F. (1978), *Phytochemistry*, **17**, 107–12.

[8] Leete, E., Lechleiter, J. C. and Carver, R. A. (1975), *Tetrahedron Lett.*, 3779–82.

[9] Keogh, M. F. and O'Donovan, D. G. (1970), *J. Chem. Soc.*, 1792–7.

[10] Gupta, R. N. and Spenser, I. D. (1967), *Can. J. Chem.*, **45**, 1275–85.

[11] Gupta, R. N. and Spenser, I. D. (1970), *Phytochemistry*, **9**, 2329–34.

[12] Leete, E. (1956), *J. Amer. Chem. Soc.*, **78**, 3520–3.

[13] Leete, E. (1969), *J. Amer. Chem. Soc.*, **91**, 1697–700.

[14] Leete, E. and Friedman, A. R. (1964), *J. Amer. Chem. Soc.*, **86**, 1224–6.

[15] Leete, E. and Chedekel, M. R. (1972), *Phytochemistry*, **11**, 2751–6.

[16] Leistner, E. and Spenser, I. D. (1973), *J. Amer. Chem. Soc.*, **95**, 4715–25.

[17] Leistner, E. and Spenser, I. D. (1975), *J. Chem. Soc. Chem. Comm.*, 378–9.

[18] Gerdes, H. J. and Leistner, E. (1979), *Phytochemistry*, **18**, 771–5.

[19] Gilbertson, T. J. (1972), *Phytochemistry*, **11**, 1737–9.

[20] Leistner, E., Gupta, R. N. and Spenser, I. D. (1973), *J. Amer. Chem. Soc.*, **95**, 4040–7.

[21] O'Donovan, D. G. and Creedon, P. B. (1971), *Tetrahedron Lett.*, 1341–4.

[22] O'Donovan, D. G., Long, D. J., Forde, E. and Geary, P. (1975), *J. Chem. Soc. Perkin I*, 415–9.

[23] Gupta, R. N. and Spenser, I. D. (1971), *Can. J. Chem.*, **49**, 384–97.

[24] Parry, R. J. (1975), *J. Chem. Soc. Chem. Comm.*, 144–5.

[25] Golobiewski, W. M., Horsewood, P. and Spenser, I. D. (1976), *J. Chem. Soc. Chem. Comm.*, 217–8.

[26] O'Donovan, D. G. and Creedon, P. B. (1974), *J. Chem. Soc. Perkin I*, 2524–8.

[27] Braekman, J.-C., Gupta, R. N., MacLean, D. B. and Spenser, I. D. (1972), *Can. J. Chem.*, **50**, 2591–602.

[28] Koo, S. H., Comer, F. and Spenser, I. D. (1970), *J. Chem. Soc. Chem. Comm.*, 897–8.

[29] Rother, A. and Schwarting, A. E. (1972), *Phytochemistry*, **11**, 2475–80.

[30] Schütte, H. R., Hindorf, H., Mothes, K. and Hübner, G. (1964), *Annalen*, **680**, 93–104.

[31] Schütte, H. R. and Hindorf, H. (1964), *Z. Naturforsch.*, **19b**, 855.

[32] Nowacki, E. K. and Waller, G. R. (1975), *Phytochemistry*, **14**, 155–9.

[33] Schütte, H. R., Nowacki, E., Kovacs, P. and Liebisch, H. W. (1963), *Arch. Pharm.*, **296**, 438–41.

[34] Cho, Y. D., Martin, R. O. and Anderson, J. N. (1971), *J. Amer. Chem. Soc.*, **93**, 2087–9.

[35] Cho, Y. D. and Martin, R. O. (1971), *Can. J. Biochem.*, **49**, 971–7.
[36] Shibata, S. and Sankawa, U. (1963), *Chem. Ind.*, 1161–2.
[37] Schütte, H. R., Lehfeldt, J. and Hindorf, H. (1965), *Annalen*, **685**, 194–99.
[38] Golebiewski, W. M. and Spenser, I. D. (1976), *J. Amer. Chem. Soc.*, **98**, 6726–8.
[39] Anet, E. F. L., Hughes, G. K. and Ritchie, E. (1949), *Austral. J. Scientific Res., Ser. 2A*, 616–21.
[40] Robinson, R. (1917), *J. Chem. Soc.*, 876–99.
[41] Leete, E. (1962), *J. Amer. Chem. Soc.*, **84**, 55–7.
[42] Leete, E. and Nelson, S. J. (1969), *Phytochemistry*, **8**, 413–8.
[43] Liebisch, H. W., Schütte, H. R. and Mothes, K. (1963), *Annalen*, **668**, 139–44.
[44] Ahmad, A. and Leete, E. (1970), *Phytochemistry*, **9**, 2345–7.
[45] Lamberts, B. L., Dewey, L. J. and Byerrum, R. U. (1959), *Biochim. Biophys. Acta*, **33**, 22–6.
[46] Leete, E., Gros, G. and Gilbertson, T. J. (1964), *Tetrahedron Lett.*, 587–92.
[47] Rueppel, M. L., Mundy, B. P. and Rapoport, H. (1974), *Phytochemistry*, **13**, 141–51.
[48] Leete, E. (1976), *J. Org. Chem.*, **41**, 3438–41.
[49] Mizusaki, S., Tanabe, Y., Noguchi, M. and Tamaki, E. (1972), *Phytochemistry*, **11**, 2757–62.
[50] Leete, E. and Liu, Y.-Y. (1973), *Phytochemistry*, **12**, 593–6.
[51] Zielke, H. R., Reinke, C. M. and Byerrum, R. U. (1969), *J. Biol. Chem.*, **244**, 95–8.
[52] O'Donovan, D. G. and Keogh, M. F. (1969), *J. Chem. Soc. (C)*, 223–6.
[53] Leete, E. (1972), *Phytochemistry*, **11**, 1713–16.
[54] Romeike, A. and Fodor, G. (1960), *Tetrahedron Lett.*, No. 22, 1–4.
[55] Leete, E. and Lucast, D. H. (1976), *Tetrahedron Lett.*, 3401–4.
[56] Leete, E., Kowanko, N. and Newmark, R. A. (1975), *J. Amer. Chem. Soc.*, **97**, 6826–30.
[57] Ansarin, M. and Woolley, J. G. (1978), *J. Pharm. Pharmacol.*, **30**, 82P.
[58] Beresford, P. J. and Woolley, J. G. (1974), *Phytochemistry*, **13**, 2143–4.
[59] Beresford, P. J. and Woolley, J. G. (1974), *Phytochemistry*, **13**, 2511–3.
[60] Leete, E. (1973), *Phytochemistry*, **12**, 2203–5.
[61] Robins, D. J., Bale, N. M. and Crout, D. H. G. (1974), *J. Chem. Soc. Perkin I*, 2082–6.
[62] Davies, N. M. and Crout, D. H. G. (1974), *J. Chem. Soc. Perkin I*, 2079–82.
[63] Robins, D. J. and Sweeney, J. R. (1979), *J. Chem. Soc. Chem. Comm.*, 120–1.
[64] Herbert, R. B., Jackson, F. B. and Nicolson, I. T. (1976), *J. Chem. Soc. Chem. Comm.*, 865–7.
[65] Herbert, R. B. and Jackson, F. B. (1977), *J. Chem. Soc. Chem. Comm.*, 955–6.
[66] Leete, E. and Marion, L. (1953), *Can. J. Chem.*, **31**, 126–8.
[67] Leete, E. and Marion, L. (1954), *Can. J. Chem.*, **32**, 646–9.
[68] Lundström, J. (1971), *Acta Pharm. Suecica*, **8**, 275–302.

[69] Basmadjian, G. P. and Paul, A. G. (1971), *Lloydia*, **34**, 91–3.

[70] Kapadia, G. J., Rao, G. S., Leete, E., Fayez, M. B. E., Vaishnav, Y. N. and Fales, H. M. (1970), *J. Amer. Chem. Soc.,* **92**, 6943–51.

[71] O'Donovan, D. G. and Barry, E. (1974), *J. Chem. Soc. Perkin I*, 2528–9.

[72] Schütte, H. R. and Seelig, G. (1969), *Annalen*, **730**, 186–90.

[73] Agurell, S., Granelli, I., Leander, K. and Rosenblom, J. (1974), *Acta Chem. Scand.*, **B28**, 1175–9.

[74] Keller, W. J. (1978), *Lloydia*, **41**, 37–42.

[75] Keller, W. J. (1979), *J. Pharm. Sci.*, **68**, 85–6.

[76] Yamasaki, K., Tamaki, T., Uzawa, S., Sankawa, U. and Shibata, S. (1973), *Phytochemistry*, **12**, 2877–82.

[77] Wilson, M. L. and Coscia, C. J. (1975), *J. Amer. Chem. Soc.,* **97**, 431–2.

[78] Battersby, A. R., Jones, R. C. F. and Kazlauskas, R. (1975), *Tetrahedron Lett.*, 1873–6.

[79] Bhakuni, D. S., Singh, A. N., Tewari, S. and Kapil, R. S. (1977), *J. Chem. Soc. Perkin I*, 1662–6.

[80] Scott, A. I., Lee, S.-L. and Hirata, T. (1978), *Heterocycles*, **11**, 159–63.

[81] Brochmann-Hanssen, E., Chen, C., Chen, C. R., Chiang, H., Leung, A. Y. and McMurtrey, K. (1975), *J. Chem. Soc. Perkin I*, 1531–7.

[82] Uprety, H., Bhakuni, D. S. and Kapil, R. S. (1975), *Phytochemistry*, **14**, 1535–7.

[83] Battersby, A. R., Sheldrake, P. W., Staunton, J. and Summers, M. C. (1977), *Bioorg. Chem.*, **6**, 43–7.

[84] Barton, D. H. R., Kirby, G. W. and Wiechers, A. (1966), *J. Chem. Soc. (C)*, 2313–9.

[85] Bhakuni, D. S., Singh, A. N. and Jain, S. (1978), *J. Chem. Soc. Perkin I*, 1318–21.

[86] Bhakuni, D. S., Singh, A. N., Jain, S. and Kapil, R. S. (1978), *J. Chem. Soc. Chem. Comm.*, 226–8.

[87] Prakash, O., Bhakuni, D. S. and Kapil, R. S. (1979), *J. Chem. Soc. Perkin I*, 1515–8.

[88] Bhakuni, D. S., Tewari, S. and Kapil, R. S. (1977), *J. Chem. Soc. Perkin I*, 706–9.

[89] Blaschke, G., Waldheim, G., von Schantz, M. and Peura, P. (1974), *Arch. Pharm.*, **307**, 122–30.

[90] Brochmann-Hanssen, E., Chen, C.-H., Chiang, H.-C. and McMurtrey, K. (1972), *J. Chem. Soc. Chem. Comm.*, 1269.

[91] Prakash, O., Bhakuni, D. S. and Kapil, R. S. (1978), *J. Chem. Soc. Perkin I*, 622–4.

[92] Battersby, A. R., Brocksom, T. J. and Ramage, R. (1969), *J. Chem. Soc. Chem. Comm.*, 464–5.

[93] Battersby, A. R., McHugh, J. L., Staunton, J. and Todd, M. (1971), *J. Chem. Soc. Chem. Comm.*, 985–6.

[94] Haynes, L. J., Stuart, K. L., Barton, D. H. R., Bhakuni, D. S. and Kirby, G. W. (1965), *J. Chem. Soc. Chem. Comm.*, 141–2.

[95] Barton, D. H. R., Bhakuni, D. S., Chapman, G. M. and Kirby, G. W. (1967), *J. Chem. Soc. (C)*, 2134–40.

[96] Bhakuni, D. S., Satish, S., Uprety, H. and Kapil, R. S. (1974), *Phytochemistry*, **13**, 2767–9.

[97] Barton, D. H. R., Bracho, R. D., Potter, C. J. and Widdowson, D. A. (1974), *J. Chem. Soc. Perkin I*, 2278–83.

[98] Bhakuni, D. S. and Singh, A. N. (1978), *J. Chem. Soc. Perkin I*, 618–2.

[99] Battersby, A. R. and Binks, R. (1960), *Proc. Chem. Soc.*, 360–1.

[100] Battersby, A. R., Binks, R., Francis, R. J., McCaldin, D. J. and Ramuz, H. (1964), *J. Chem. Soc.*, 3600–10.

[101] Battersby, A. R., Foulkes, D. M. and Binks, R. (1965), *J. Chem. Soc.*, 3323–32.

[102] Borkowski, P. R., Horn, J. S. and Rapoport, H. (1978), *J. Amer. Chem. Soc.*, **100**, 276–81.

[103] Parker, H. I., Blaschke, G. and Rapoport, H. (1972), *J. Amer. Chem. Soc.*, **94**, 1276–82.

[104] Battersby, A. R. and Harper, B. J. T. (1960), *Tetrahedron Lett.*, No. 27, pp. 21–4.

[105] Horn, J. S., Paul, A. G. and Rapoport, H. (1978), *J. Amer. Chem. Soc.*, **100**, 1895–8.

[106] Battersby, A. R., Minta, A., Ottridge, A. P. and Staunton, J. (1977), *Tetrahedron Lett.*, 1321–4.

[107] Barton, D. H. R., Hesse, R. H. and Kirby, G. W. (1965), *J. Chem. Soc.*, 6379–89.

[108] Battersby, A. R., Francis, R. J., Hirst, M. and Staunton, J. (1963), *Proc. Chem. Soc.*, 268.

[109] Battersby, A. R., Francis, R. J., Hirst, M., Ruveda, E. A. and Staunton, J. (1975), *J. Chem. Soc. Perkin I*, 1140–7.

[110] Battersby, A. R., Staunton, J., Wiltshire, H. R., Bircher, B. J. and Fuganti, C. (1975), *J. Chem. Soc. Perkin I*, 1162–71.

[111] Battersby, A. R., Staunton, J., Wiltshire, H. R., Francis, R. J. and Southgate, R. (1975), *J. Chem. Soc. Perkin I*, 1147–56.

[112] Battersby, A. R., Staunton, J., Summers, M. C. and Southgate, R. (1979), *J. Chem. Soc. Perkin. I*, 45–52.

[113] Takao, N., Iwasa, K., Kamigauchi, M. and Sugiura, M. (1976), *Chem. and Pharm. Bull. (Japan)*, **24**, 2859–68.

[114] Holland, H. L., Castillo, M., MacLean, D. B. and Spenser, I. D. (1974), *Can. J. Chem.*, **52**, 2818–31.

[115] Rönsch, H. (1977), *Phytochemistry*, **16**, 691–8.

[116] Tani, C. and Tagahara, K. (1977), *J. Pharm. Soc. Japan*, **97**, 93–102 (for the closely related alkaloid, rhoeadine).

[117] Battersby, A. R., Dobson, T. A., Foulkes, D. M. and Herbert, R. B. (1972), *J. Chem. Soc. Perkin I*, 1730–6.

[118] Battersby, A. R., Herbert, R. B., Pijewska, L. Santavý, F. and Sedmera, P. (1972), *J. Chem. Soc. Perkin I*, 1736–40.

[119] Battersby, A. R., Herbert, R. B., McDonald, E., Ramage, R. and Clements, J. H. (1972), *J. Chem. Soc. Perkin I*, 1972, 1741–6.

[120] Battersby, A. R., Sheldrake, P. W. and Milner, J. A. (1974), *Tetrahedron Lett.*, 3315–8.

[121] Barker, A. C., Battersby, A. R., McDonald, E., Ramage, R. and Clements, J. H. (1967), *J. Chem. Soc. Chem. Comm.*, 390–2.

[122] Battersby, A. R., Böhler, P., Munro, M. H. G. and Ramage R. (1974), *J. Chem. Soc. Perkin I*, 1399–402.

[123] Battersby, A. R., McDonald, E., Milner, J. A., Johns, S. R.,

Lamberton, J. A. and Sioumis, A. A. (1975), *Tetrahedron Lett.*, 3419–22.

[124] Schwab, J. M., Chang, M. N. T. and Parry, R. J. (1977), *J. Amer. Chem. Soc.*, **99**, 2368–70.

[125] Battersby, A. R., Binks, R., Breuer, S. W., Fales, H. M., Wildman, W. C. and Highet, R. J. (1964), *J. Chem. Soc.*, 1595–609.

[126] Zulalian, J. and Suhadolnik, R. J. (1964), *Proc. Chem. Soc.*, 422–3.

[127] Wightman, R. H., Staunton, J., Battersby, A. R. and Hanson, K. R. (1972), *J. Chem. Soc. Perkin I*, 2355–64.

[128] Barton, D. H. R., Kirby, G. W., Taylor, J. B. and Thomas, G. M. (1963), *J. Chem. Soc.*, 4545–58.

[129] Bennett, D. J. and Kirby, G. W. (1968), *J. Chem. Soc. (C)*, 442–6.

[130] Leete, E. and Louden, M. C. L. (1968), *J. Amer. Chem. Soc.*, **90**, 6837–41.

[131] O'Donovan, D. G. and Horan, H. (1971), *J. Chem. Soc. (C)*, 331–4.

[132] Kirby, G. W. and Tiwari, H. P. (1966), *J. Chem. Soc. (C)*, 676–82.

[133] Fuganti, C. (1969), *Chim. Ind. (Milan)*, **51**, 1254–5.

[134] Fales, H. M., Mann, J. and Mudd, S. H. (1963), *J. Amer. Chem. Soc.*, **85**, 2025–6.

[135] Bhandarkar, J. G. and Kirby, G. W. (1970), *J. Chem. Soc. (C)*, 1224–7.

[136] Fuganti, C., Ghiringhelli, D. and Grasselli, P. (1974), *J. Chem. Soc. Chem. Comm.*, 350–1.

[137] Fuganti, C. and Mazza, M. (1972), *J. Chem. Soc. Chem. Comm.*, 936–7.

[138] Bruce, I. T. and Kirby, G. W. (1968), *J. Chem. Soc. Chem. Comm.*, 207–8.

[139] Battersby, A. R., Kelsey, J. W., Staunton, J. and Suckling, K. E. (1973), *J. Chem. Soc. Perkin I*, 1609–15.

[140] Kirby, G. W. and Michael, J. (1973), *J. Chem. Soc. Perkin I*, 115–20.

[141] Fuganti, C. and Mazza, M. (1971), *J. Chem. Soc. Chem. Comm.*, 1196–7.

[142] Fuganti, C. and Mazza, M. (1973), *J. Chem. Soc. Perkin I*, 954–6.

[143] Fuganti, C. (1973), *Gazzetta*, **103**, 1255–8.

[144] Fuganti, C. and Mazza, M. (1972), *J. Chem. Soc. Chem. Comm.*, 239.

[145] Fuganti, C. (1973), *Tetrahedron Lett.*, 1785–8.

[146] Fuganti, C., Ghiringhelli, D. and Grasselli, P. (1973), *J. Chem. Soc. Chem. Comm.*, 430–1.

[147] Feinstein, A. I. and Wildman, W. C. (1976), *J. Org. Chem.*, **41**, 2447–50.

[148] Jeffs, P. W., Campbell, H. F., Farrier, D. S., Ganguli, G., Martin, N. H. and Molina, G. (1974), *Phytochemistry*, **13**, 933–45.

[149] Jeffs, P. W., Johnson, D. B., Martin, N. H. and Rauckman, B. S. (1976), *J. Chem. Soc. Chem. Comm.*, 82–3.

[150] Jeffs, P. W., Karle, J. M. and Martin, N. H. (1978), *Phytochemistry*, **17**, 719–28.

[151] Munsche, D. and Mothes, K. (1965), *Phytochemistry*, **4**, 705–12.

[152] Schröder, P. and Luckner, M. (1966), *Pharmazie*, **21**, 642.

[153] Tipton, C. L., Wang, M.-C., Tsao, F. H.-C., Tu, C. L. and Husted, R. R. (1973), *Phytochemistry*, **12**, 347–52.

[154] Blaschke-Cobet, M. and Luckner, M. (1973), *Phytochemistry*, **12**, 2393–8.

[155] Johne, S., Waiblinger, K. and Gröger, D. (1970), *Eur. J. Biochem.*, **15**, 415–20.

[156] O'Donovan, D. G. and Horan, H. (1970), *J. Chem. Soc. (C)*, 2466–70.

[157] Yamazaki, M., Ikuta, A., Mori, T. and Kawana, T. (1967), *Tetrahedron Lett.*, 3317–20.

[158] Prager, R. H. and Thedgold, H. M. (1969), *Austral. J. Chem.*, **22**, 2627–34.

[159] Gröger, D. and Johne, S. (1968), *Z. Naturforsch.*, **23b**, 1072–5.

[160] Liljegren, D. R. (1971), *Phytochemistry*, **10**, 2661–9.

[161] Waiblinger, K., Johne, S. and Gröger, D. (1972), *Phytochemistry*, **11**, 2263–5.

[162] Waiblinger, K., Johne, S. and Gröger, D. (1973), *Pharmazie*, **28**, 403–6.

[163] Grundon, M. F., Harrison, D. M. and Spyropoulos, C. G. (1975), *J. Chem. Soc. Perkin I*, 302–4.

[164] Boulanger, D., Bailey, B. K. and Steck, W. (1973), *Phytochemistry*, **12**, 2399–405.

[165] Leete, E. and Minich, M. L. (1977), *Phytochemistry*, **16**, 149–50.

[166] Agurell, S. and Nilsson, J. L. G. (1968), *Acta Chem. Scand.*, **22**, 1210–18.

[167] Baxter, C. and Slaytor, M. (1972), *Phytochemistry*, **11**, 2767–73.

[168] McFarlane, I. J. and Slaytor, M. (1972), *Phytochemistry*, **11**, 229–34.

[169] O'Donovan, D. G. and Keogh, M. F. (1966), *J. Chem. Soc. (C)*, 1570–2.

[170] Battersby, A. R., Burnett, A. R. and Parsons, P. G. (1969), *J. Chem. Soc. (C)*, 1193–200.

[171] Wenkert, E. (1962), *J. Amer. Chem. Soc.*, **84**, 98–102.

[172] Thomas, R. (1961), *Tetrahedron Lett.*, 544–53.

[173] Battersby, A. R., Hall, E. S. and Southgate, R. (1969), *J. Chem. Soc. (C)*, 721–8.

[174] Battersby, A. R., Byrne, J. C., Kapil, R. S., Martin, J. A., Payne, T. G., Arigoni, D. and Loew, P. (1968), *J. Chem. Soc. Chem. Comm.*, 951–3.

[175] Escher, S., Loew, P. and Arigoni, D. (1970), *J. Chem. Soc. Chem. Comm.*, 823–5 (and following two papers).

[176] Battersby, A. R., Burnett, A. R. and Parsons, R. G. (1969), *J. Chem. Soc. (C)*, 1187–92.

[177] Rueffer, M., Nagakura, N. and Zenk, M. H. (1978), *Tetrahedron Lett.*, 1593–6.

[178] Battersby, A. R., Lewis, N. G. and Tippett, J. M. (1978), *Tetrahedron Lett.*, 4849–52.

[179] Scott, A. I., Lee, S.-L. and Wan, W. (1977), *Biochem. Biophys. Res. Comm.*, **75**, 1004–9.

[180] Stöckigt, J., Husson, H. P., Kan-Fan, C. and Zenk, M. H. (1977), *J. Chem. Soc. Chem. Comm.*, 164–6.

[181] Stöckigt, J., Rueffer, M., Zenk, M. H. and Hoyer, G.-A. (1978), *Planta Med.*, **33**, 188–92.

[182] Heimberger, S. I. and Scott, A. I. (1973), *J. Chem. Soc. Chem. Comm.*, 217–8.

[183] Battersby, A. R. and Hall, E. S. (1969), *J. Chem. Soc. Chem. Comm.*, 793–4.

[184] Scott, A. I., Cherry, P. C. and Qureshi, A. A. (1969), *J. Amer. Chem. Soc.*, **91**, 4932–3.

[185] Stöckigt, J. (1978), *J. Chem. Soc. Chem. Comm.*, 1097–9.

[186] Scott, A. I., Reichardt, P. B., Slaytor, M. B. and Sweeney, J. G. (1971), *Bioorg. Chem.*, **1**, 157–73.

[187] Kutney, J. P., Beck, J. F., Eggers, N. J., Hanssen, H. W., Sood, R. S. and Westcott, N. D. (1971), *J. Amer. Chem. Soc.*, **93**, 7322–4.

[188] Scott, A. I., Gueritte, F. and Lee, S.-L. (1978), *J. Amer. Chem. Soc.*, **100**, 6253–5.

[189] Stuart, K. L., Kutney, J. P., Honda, T. and Worth, B. R. (1978), *Heterocycles*, **9**, 1419–27.

[190] Kutney, J. P., Beck, J. F., Nelson, V. R. and Sood, R. S. (1971), *J. Amer. Chem. Soc.*, **93**, 255–7.

[191] Kutney, J. P., Beck, J. F., Ehret, C., Poulton, G., Sood, R. S. and Westcott, N. D. (1971), *Bioorg. Chem.*, **1**, 194–206.

[192] Battersby, A. R. and Parry, R. J. (1971), *J. Chem. Soc. Chem. Comm.*, 31–2.

[193] Hutchinson, C. R., Heckendorf, A. H., Daddona, P. E., Hagaman, E. and Wenkert, E. (1974), *J. Amer. Chem. Soc.*, **96**, 5609–11.

[194] Sheriha, G. M. and Rapoport, H. (1976), *Phytochemistry*, **15**, 505–8.

[195] Nagakura, N., Höfle, G. and Zenk, M. H. (1978), *J. Chem. Soc. Chem. Comm.*, 896–8.

[196] Nagakura, N., Höfle, G., Coggiola, D. and Zenk, M. H. (1978), *Planta Med.*, **34**, 381–9.

[197] Horan, H. and O'Donovan, D. G. (1971), *J. Chem. Soc. (C)*, 2083–5.

[198] Rosenberg, H. and Paul, A. G. (1972), *Lloydia*, **34**, 372–6.

[199] Leete, E. and Bodem, G. B. (1973), *J. Chem. Soc. Chem. Comm.*, 522–3.

[200] Fischer, N. and Dreiding, A. S. (1972), *Helv. Chim. Acta*, **55**, 649–58.

[201] Impellizzeri, G. and Piattelli, M. (1972), *Phytochemistry*, **11**, 2499–502.

7. Microbial metabolites containing nitrogen

7.1 Introduction

There is a wide variety of metabolites containing nitrogen, which is produced by micro-organisms. The nitrogen atom (or atoms) most frequently is derived ultimately from an α-amino acid which also provides at least part of the carbon skeleton. Modifications to cyclic dipeptides are commonly encountered as secondary metabolites (Sections 7.3 and 7.4). In the case of the vastly important pharmaceuticals, the penicillins and cephalosporins (Section 7.6.5), a linear tripeptide is involved in biosynthesis.

Tryptophan (7.25) serves as a precursor for a number of microbial metabolites. A notable example is the ergot alkaloids (Section 7.5.1). Other aromatic amino acids are involved in the biosynthesis of various metabolites. Their origins are through shikimic acid (7.78) (see Section 5.1). Shikimic acid itself, or a close metabolic relative, serves as a source for some metabolites, e.g. phenazines (Section 7.5.5) and the ansamycins (Section 7.6.1). For compounds like the latter, acetate and propionate are also important starting materials for biosynthesis. Another important part source for many metabolites is mevalonate, invariably as a C_5 (dimethylallyl) unit.

7.2 Piperidine and pyridine metabolites

† Pipecolic acid (7.1) occurs widely in plants, animals and micro-organisms. It has been found, in representative species of each, to derive from lysine with the D-isomer preferred (see Section 6.2.1; Scheme 6.9). Slaframine (7.5), a toxin produced by the fungus, *Rhizoctonia leguminicola*, has been firmly shown to be a pipecolic acid (7.1) metabolite. Results of experiments with likely precursors have allowed definition of the pathway shown in Scheme 7.1. This is supported by the discovery that a cell-free extract of *R. leguminicola* would catalyse the NADPH-dependent transformation of (7.2) into (7.3), and also the conversion of (7.4) into slaframine (7.5) in the presence of acetyl-CoA. Lysine is a precursor but curiously, in contrast to the evidence on pipecolic acid mentioned above (see also Section 6.2.1), the L-isomer is preferred over its antipode [2].

(7.1)   (7.2)   (7.3)

(7.5) Slaframine   (7.4)

Scheme 7.1

† Two possible primary metabolic pathways lead to lysine in different organisms [1]. An intermediate in one of these routes is dihy-drodipicolinic acid (7.6). In *Bacillus megaterium* this is the point at which diversion to a secondary product, dipicolinic acid (7.7), may occur [3]. In the unrelated organism *Penicillium citreo-viride*, dipicolinic acid appears to be formed by diversion from the other route to lysine [4].

(7.6)   (7.7) Dipicolinic acid

† By contrast, the biosynthesis of nigrifactin (7.8) is by linear combi-nation of six acetate units. In this it resembles the plant alkaloid coni-ine (Section 6.2.1; Scheme 6.5), and a further resemblance is seen in the apparent implication of (7.9) and (7.10) as intermediates. The compounds (7.11) and (7.12), plausibly lying on the biosynthetic pathway between (7.10) and nigrifactin (7.8), have also been found to be precursors for (7.8) [5].

(7.8) Nigrifactin

(7.9) R = CO₂H
(7.10) R = CHO   (7.11)   (7.12)

† Three pyridine metabolites, fusaric acid (7.13), proferrorosamine A (7.16) and tenellin (7.18), have been found to have disparate origins. Fusaric acid (7.13) derives from acetate (side-chain plus C-5 and C-6) and aspartic acid (7.14) (C-2, C-3, and C-4 plus the carboxy-group), and its origins thus resemble the biosynthesis of nicotinic acid from precursors other than tryptophan (Section 6.2.2; Scheme 6.16) [6].

(7.13) Fusaric acid   (7.14)   (7.15)   (7.16) Proferrorosamine A

The picolonic part [as (7.15)] of proferrorosamine A (7.16) originates in lysine (and glutamic acid), being formed via picolinic acid (7.15) [7].

† The biosynthesis of the fungal metabolite tenellin (7.18), has been studied in some detail [8, 9]. Notable use of ^{13}C-labelled precursors gave results which establish the origins of this metabolite as those shown in (7.18); the intact acetate units indicated follow in the usual way (Section 2.2.2) from experiments with [1,2-^{13}C$_2$]acetate. It is to be noted that the branched side chain originates from acetate plus methyl groups from methionine, rather than from the alternative, propionate, which is implicated in the biosynthesis of pyrindicin (7.19) [10], a *Streptomyces* metabolite. Incorporation of phenylalanine (7.17)

(7.17) Phenylalanine   (7.18) Tenellin   Methionine (■)

CH$_3$ — CO$_2$H

CH$_3$-CH$_2$-CO$_2$H

(7.19) Pyrindicin

into (7.18) is with rearrangement of the side-chain (C-1 of the amino acid appears at C-4 of tenellin, and C-2 at C-6). This is the same reordering of atoms as seen in tropic acid biosynthesis (Section 6.2.2; Scheme 6.18) and it has been shown to involve a similar intramolecular 1,2-shift of the phenylalanine carboxy-group (see Section 6.2.2 for a more detailed discussion). The two final products, tropic acid and (7.18), are manifestly dissimilar and the fact that one is fungal and the other of plant origin, argue that the rearrangement is one which is closely related to phenylalanine metabolism rather than formation of (7.18) or tropic acid.

† Phomazarin (7.20) has been shown by use of [^{13}C]-labelled precursors to be formed from a single polyketide chain of nine intact acetate units [see (7.20)] with C-15 as the (only) starter acetate (see Section

(7.20) Phomazarin   (7.21)

3.2.1 for further discussion of 'starter' acetate). Nitrogen intercalates in this chain at some point in biosynthesis, and the substrate for this is suggested to be (7.21) [11].

7.3   Diketopiperazines [12]

A variety of metabolites, isolated from fungi or actinomycetes, displays a diketopiperazine ring [as (7.22)] in modified form, e.g. echinulin (7.24). (A related system is found in the benzodiazepines, see below.) The diketopiperazine metabolites can be seen as arising by combination of two α-amino acid residues through amide (peptide) linkages; in the case of echinulin these amino acids are tryptophan (7.25) and alanine (7.26), and the diketopiperazine (7.22) is also a precursor for (7.24).

(7.22) R = H
(7.23) R = $\times$ Me, Me

(7.24) Echinulin

The remaining, obviously isoprenoid, atoms in echinulin have been shown to arise from mevalonate in *Aspergillus* sp., as expected. Dimethylallyl pyrophosphate would follow as the source of the three isoprenoid residues and it has been found that a partially purified enzyme preparation from *A. amstelodami* would catalyse the transfer of an isoprene unit from dimethylallyl pyrophosphate (7.27) to (7.22) to yield (7.23); this compound was then found to be an intact precursor for echinulin (7.24). Prenylation of C-2 thus occurs before prenylation of the other two sites in echinulin biosynthesis [13, 14].

A similar pathway is deduced to lead to brevianamide A (7.30), in *Penicillium brevicompactum*, from tryptophan (7.25) and proline through the diketopiperazine (7.28), which has been isolated from *P. brevicompactum*. A further intermediate may be the *Aspergillus ustus* metabolite (7.29) (cf. echinulin biosynthesis) [15].

(7.25) Tryptophan

(7.26) Alanine

(7.27)

(7.28) R = H
(7.29) R = $\times$ Me, Me

(7.30) Brevianamide A

Mycelianamide (7.32) is a diketopiperazine formed from tyrosine (7.31) rather than tryptophan. However, the appropriate

(7.31) Tyrosine   (7.32) Mycelianamide

diketopiperazines, *cyclo*-(L-alanyl-L-tyrosyl) and *cyclo*-(L-alanyl-D-tyrosyl), with radioactive labels, failed to act as precursors, suggesting possibly that the diketopiperazine when formed remains enzyme bound until after further reaction, and no equilibration occurs with unbound (radioactive) diketopiperazine [16].

† The desaturation of the tyrosine residue in mycelianamide (7.32) has been shown, with tyrosine samples chirally tritiated at C-3, to involve *cis* removal of hydrogen from L-tyrosine [17]. A (Z)-double bond similar to that in (7.32) is present in an echinulin (7.24) relative, and the desaturation proceeds again in the same stereochemical sense [13, 14].

† Pulcheriminic acid (7.33) is, like mycelianamide, an *N,N*-dihydroxydiketopiperazine. It has been concluded that it derives by hydroxylation of the diketopiperazine (7.34) formed from two molecules of leucine [18].

(7.33) R = OH
(7.34) R = H

† Other simple diketopiperazines examined are rhodotorulic and dimeric acids [19, 20], and roquefortine (7.35) [21]. Deuteriated tryptophan gave roquefortine (7.35) in which deuterium at C-2′ [≡ C-5a in (7.35)] was lost. This indicates that the C_5 isoprene unit at C-10b of (7.35) may have arrived at this site via C-5a, with (7.36) as a possible intermediate [cf. echinulin (7.24) above].

(7.35) Roquefortine   (7.36)

Gliotoxin (7.39) is unusual amongst diketopiperazine metabolites in having a disulphide bridge. Its biosynthesis though proceeds through a diketopiperazine [*cyclo*-(L-phenylalanyl-L-seryl) (7.37)]; the precursor amino acids are serine and phenylalanine (7.17). [Ar-$^2H_5$]phenylalanine was incorporated into gliotoxin with retention of all five deuterium atoms. This excludes aromatic hydroxy-intermediates, and biosynthesis has very reasonably been suggested to proceed via the arene oxide (7.38), as shown in Scheme 7.2 [22]. A

(7.37)
(7.38)
(7.39) Gliotoxin
(7.40)

Scheme 7.2

similar pathway leads to (7.40), ring expansion from an intermediate benzenoid ring being plausibly associated with another arene oxide (7.41). (For further discussion of arene oxides, see Section 1.3.2.)

(7.41)

(7.42) Sporidesmin

† Sporidesmin (7.42) is also a dithiodiketopiperazine. It derives from tryptophan and alanine; the hydroxy group at C-3 [≡ C-3 in tryptophan (7.25)] enters with normal retention of configuration [23]. An intriguing problem relates to the entry of sulphur into this and other metabolites above: the mechanism is unknown.

7.4 Benzodiazepines

The benzodiazepines, e.g. cyclopenin (7.46), are, formally at least, related to the diketopiperazines in being formed from two amino acids. For cyclopenin (7.46) and cyclopenol (7.47), in *Penicillium cyclopium*, they are anthranilic acid (7.43) and phenylalanine (7.17). The first detectable intermediates are cyclopeptine (7.44) and dehydrocyclopeptine (7.45), which are interconvertible; earlier intermediates apparently only exist enzyme-bound, not being equilibrated with fed precursors.

The epoxide and aromatic oxygens arise from molecular oxygen, and an enzyme which will effect the unusual aromatic *meta*-hydroxylation of cyclopenin (7.46) to give cyclopenol (7.47) has been isolated from *P. cyclopium*. It shows typical mixed-function oxidase properties, requiring both oxygen and a hydrogen donating cofactor.

Also found in *P. cyclopium* cultures are viridicatin (7.48) and viridicatol (7.49). They are enzymically derived from cyclopenin (7.46) and cyclopenol (7.47), respectively, and the peculiar rearrangement is catalysed in a similar way by base or acid [17, 24].

Although anthramycin (7.50) can be seen to contain a modified

(7.43) Anthranilic acid + Phenylalanine (7.17) → (7.44) ⇌ (7.45)

(7.48) R=H
(7.49) R=OH

(7.47) Cyclopenol

(7.46) Cyclopenin

Scheme 7.3

anthranilic acid moiety (4-methyl-3-hydroxyanthranilic acid; proved to have the expected origins in tryptophan, cf. actinomycin biosynthesis, below) the origin of the remaining atoms (C_8N unit) is not obvious. Results have been obtained which show, however, that this C_8 unit originates in tyrosine [and dopa (7.51)]. Incorporation of tyrosine (7.31) was with retention of seven of the nine carbon atoms and the eighth carbon (C-14) derived from the methyl group of methionine.

(7.50) Anthramycin

Evidence on the mechanism of fragmentation of the tyrosine/dopa aromatic ring comes from experiments with tyrosine labelled at C-3′ and C-5′ with tritium or deuterium. Conversion of tyrosine (7.31) into dopa (7.51) inevitably means loss of half of the label. Of three pathways leading from dopa to anthramycin (7.50) one (Scheme 7.4)

Tyrosine (7.31) → (7.51) → Methionine (Me•)

Scheme 7.4

results in deuterium/tritium retention (at C-13), and two in loss of the label. Retention of half the tyrosine label in anthramycin (in the case of deuterium proved to reside at C-13) [25] establishes the route (a) outlined in Scheme 7.4.

† A related biosynthesis has been found for related metabolites: 11-demethyltomaymycin and lincomycin [25, 26].

7.5   Metabolites derived from tryptophan pathway

This section is concerned with diverse metabolites based on tryptophan (some also appear above). A large group is constituted by the ergot alkaloids.

7.5.1   Ergot alkaloids [27]

Ergot alkaloids, e.g. elymoclavine (7.55), are produced by a fungus, *Claviceps purpurea*, which infects rye and other grasses. They have been extensively studied and there are several fascinating aspects of their biosynthesis.

An impressive body of evidence has established that these 'alkaloids'* are formed from L-tryptophan (7.25) which condenses at C-4' with dimethylallyl pyrophosphate (7.27), derived in the usual way from (3-*R*)-mevalonic acid, to give dimethylallyltryptophan (7.52) [28]; this is then modified to give, e.g. elymoclavine (7.55). The main biosynthetic pathway is (7.52) → chanoclavine-I (7.53) → agroclavine (7.54) → elymoclavine (7.55) → lysergic acid (7.56) [27].

(7.52)   (7.53) Chanoclavine-I   (7.54) Agroclavine   (7.55) Elymoclavine
Scheme 7.5

Most interestingly it has been found that the conversion of (7.52) through (7.53) into (7.54) and (7.55) involves two enigmatic changes in the ordering of the methyl groups about the double bond in (7.52) [29] (trace the labels ▲ and ● through the various compounds, Scheme 7.5); and it is logical to associate these isomerizations with the actual ring-closure reactions. The mechanism for closing ring C [formation of (7.53)] is unknown and the timing of the necessary allylic hydroxylation is uncertain. But the formation of ring D and associated reactions can be accounted for satisfactorily [30]. In the conversion of chanoclavine-1 (7.53) into elymoclavine (7.55) one of the

---

*The term alkaloid only properly applies to bases isolated from plants.

C-17 hydrogens is lost; the other appears at C-7 as expected. This suggested that the aldehyde (7.57) might be an intermediate. This received strong support when radioactive (7.57) was shown to be a

(7.56) Lysergic acid   (7.57)   (7.58) Rugulovasine

precursor for agroclavine (7.54) and elymoclavine (7.55); a tritium label from C-17 in the precursor appeared at C-7 in (7.55). Moreover, two deuterium atoms from a sample of mevalonic acid, labelled at C-3′ were retained on formation of chanoclavine-I (C-3′ of mevalonate becomes C-17 of chanoclavine-I); only one of these was retained into elymoclavine (7.55), consistent with the intermediacy of the aldehyde (7.57). Further, the retained deuterium atom (at C-7) was largely equatorial in (7.55) indicating proton addition to (7.57) would be stereospecific.

In considering the ring-closure of (7.53) to give (7.54) and the apparently connected double-bond isomerization, knowledge of the fate of the proton at C-9 in (7.53) is important. It was found to be incompletely retained (~70%) during biosynthesis (that at C-10 is completely retained). In an experiment with a 1:1 mixture of [2-^{13}C]- and [4-^{2}H$_2$]-mevalonate, the derived (7.53) showed the expected mixture of singly labelled species, but the elymoclavine (7.55) showed an appreciable percentage of double-labelled molecules, i.e. molecules which contained both ^{13}C and deuterium. These results and the required double-bond isomerization are neatly accounted for in terms of the mechanism shown in Scheme 7.6 [30] in which there is an

(7.54)

Scheme 7.6

inter-molecular shift of the C-9 proton (hence the formation of doubly labelled elymoclavine). In the proposed sequence the aldehyde group is masked to allow anti-Michael addition of Enz-X-H to the double bond. Rotation around the 8,9-bond allows transfer of the original C-9 hydrogen to the enzyme in the subsequent elimination step. Assuming slow exchange of the hydrogen attached to the enzyme, most of it would be transferred to a molecule of (7.57) in the next cycle [because of dilution in the culture by unlabelled species, (7.57) might, or might not be, labelled].

Rugulovasine (7.58) and related *Penicillium* metabolites are biosynthesized via dimethylallyltryptophan (7.52) but not chanoclavine-I (7.53) [31]. Of considerable interest is the finding that ergot alkaloids are elaborated by higher plants, also from tryptophan and mevalonic acid [32].

Lysergic acid (7.56), formed from elymoclavine (7.55), is a precursor for a range of peptidic ergot bases, e.g. ergotamine (7.59).

(7.59) Ergotamine

Although the expected amino acids are incorporated into the complex peptidic alkaloids, attempts to obtain incorporation of larger fragments have met with little success and it is currently believed that assembly of the alkaloids from lysergic acid and the relevant amino acids occurs without desorption from an enzyme surface at any point or equilibration with exogenous (fed) material [33, 34].

7.5.2 Cyclopiazonic acid

† α-Cyclopiazonic acid (7.62) is formed in *Penicillium cyclopium* from tryptophan, mevalonate, and an acetate-derived C_4 unit [heavy bonding in (7.62)] by way of β-cyclopiazonic acid (7.61). An earlier intermediate is (7.60). [The ergot precursor, dimethylallyltryptophan (7.52) was not incorporated.]

(7.60)   (7.61)   (7.62) α-Cyclopiazonic acid

† Tritium label at C-3 of tryptophan (*7.25*) is retained as far as (*7.61*), and subsequent conversion into (*7.62*) involves stereospecific removal of the tryptophan (3-*pro-S*)-proton. It follows from this, and the stereochemistry of (*7.62*), that C–C bond formation within (*7.61*) takes place from the opposite side of the molecule to proton removal. The retention of label from [2-³H]tryptophan [label at C-5 of (*7.62*)] indicates that bond formation to C-4 cannot involve a 4,5-dehydro-intermediate, but an intermediate with a double bond 1,4 is still possible [35].

7.5.3 Indolmycin

Indolmycin (*7.66*), a *Streptomyces griseus* metabolite, is derived as shown in Scheme 7.7 [36]. Of particular interest is the *C*-methylation at what is C-3 in tryptophan (*7.25*). Mechanistically indolepyruvic acid (*7.63*) is an

Scheme 7.7

attractive substrate for methylation via the enol (*7.64*) and enzymes have been isolated which will catalyse (*7.25*) → (*7.63*) and (*7.64*) → (*7.65*) (Scheme 7.7); removal of a tryptophan C-3 proton is stereospecific (*pro-R* proton) which indicates a stereospecific enolization reaction. Transfer of a methyl group from *S*-adenosyl-methionine to (*7.64*) occurs with inversion of configuration [36].

7.5.4 Streptonigrin and pyrrolnitrin

Streptonigrin (*7.67*) is a *Streptomyces flocculus* metabolite. It has been shown to have its genesis in part from tryptophan (via 3-methyltryptophan) (rings C and D). A notable point is the clever use of ¹³C–¹⁵N coupling: observation of this coupling in (*7.67*) derived from [2′-¹³C, ¹⁵N₁′,]tryptophan indicates both atoms are retained and that the necessary cleavage of tryptophan occurs along the dotted line as shown [37]. It is to be noted that this cleavage differs from the equally unique one in pyrrolnitrin (*7.70*).

Pyrrolnitrin (*7.70*), a *Pseudomonas aureofaciens* metabolite, is formed from tryptophan with loss only of the carboxy-group in a biosynthetic sequence which obviously involves fracture of the indole nucleus. The

(7.67) Streptonigrin

(7.70) Pyrrolnitrin   (7.69)   (7.68)

proposed route is indicated by the results of feeding experiments and in part by the natural occurrence of (7.68) and (7.69) [25, 38, 39].

7.5.5 Pseudans, phenoxazinones, phenazines, and chloramphenicol

† A *Pseudomonas* sp. elaborates the pseudans, which are a group of simple quinoline derivatives with aliphatic side chains of varying length (C_7–C_{12}), e.g. pseudan-VII (7.71). The skeleton is accounted for by anthranilic acid (7.43), acetate and malonate, labelling by acetate and malonate being consistent with that expected for a fatty acid unit. Since 4-hydroxy-2-quinolone, a plant quinoline alkaloid precursor, was not incorporated it follows that (7.71) is assembled from anthranilic acid and the complete fatty acid, which its incorporation establishes as 3-oxodecanoic acid for pseudan-VII [40].

(7.71) Pseudan-VII   (7.72) R = H   (7.74) Xanthommatin
(7.73) R = OH

† The insect ommochromes, e.g. xanthommatin (7.74), derive from the products of tryptophan catabolism, kynurenine (7.72) and hydroxy-kynurenine (7.73) [41] as do the *Streptomyces antibioticus* phenox-azinones, the actinomycins (7.76). A further intermediate in the biosynthesis of (7.76) is 3-hydroxy-4-methylanthranilic acid (7.75) (cf.

(7.75)

2 x

(7.76) R = peptide, Actinomycin
(7.77) R = OH

anthramycin biosynthesis, Section 7.4), and aromatic methylation occurs on 3-hydroxykynurenine (7.73). Oxidative dimerization of (7.75) using a crude enzyme preparation from *S. antibioticus* gave actinocinin (7.77) [42].

† It might be expected from the foregoing that bacterial phenazines, e.g. phenazine-1,6-dicarboxylic acid (7.81) and phenazine-1-carboxylic acid (7.82), would derive from two molecules of anthranilic acid (7.43), but it has been proved that not only is this amino acid not involved, but also, using mutants, that biosynthesis along the pathway to aromatic amino acids gets no further than chorismic acid (7.79) (Section 5.1). An earlier intermediate on this pathway, shikimic

(7.78) Shikimic acid   (7.79) Chorismic acid   (7.80)   (7.81)

acid (7.78), is, unlike chorismic acid, assimilated into phenazines when fed to bacterial cultures. It has been used to prove the orientation of precursor units in the phenazines. In particular, [2-^{2}H]shikimic acid [as (7.78)] gave iodinin (7.84), some molecules of which were dilabelled. This proved that two molecules of shikimic acid were involved in phenazine biosynthesis. These deuterium atoms were, moreover, located at C-2 and C-7, which established, in conjunction with ^{14}C data, that the orientation of shikimic acid units is as shown in (7.80). This leads to phenazine-1,6-dicarboxylic acid (7.81) as the first phenazine to be formed and it has been shown to be a precursor for some phenazines at least (proof that it is universally a phenazine precursor is still outstanding) [43, 44].

† Common reactions found in phenazine biosynthesis are hydroxylation, as in iodinin (7.84) biosynthesis, and this may be associated with concomitant decarboxylation through (7.85) (solid arrows); iodinin

(7.82) R = H
(7.83) R = OH

(7.84)

(7.85)

(7.86)   (7.87) Pyocyanin   (7.88)

(7.91)   (7.90) Chloramphenicol   (7.89)

(*7.84*) is apparently formed in this way from (*7.86*) [45]. The latter compound does not derive from phenazine-1-carboxylic acid (*7.82*) but has an independent genesis presumably from phenazine-1,6-dicarboxylic acid (*7.81*) again via a hydroxylative decarboxylation. It is proved using deuterium-labelled precursors that pyocyanin (*7.87*) derives in a similar way from (*7.82*) via (*7.88*); enzyme-catalysed nucleophilic substitution of (*7.88*) by ammonia gives aeruginosin A (*7.89*). Opening of (*7.85*) derived from (*7.82*) without decarboxylation (broken arrows) gives 2-hydroxyphenazine-1-carboxylic acid (*7.83*) [46].

† Shikimic acid (*7.78*), rather than aromatic amino acids, is involved in chloramphenicol (*7.90*) biosynthesis via chorismic acid (*7.79*) and (*7.91*) [47].

7.6 Miscellaneous metabolites

7.6.1 *Mitomycins and ansamycins*

† There are a number of complex metabolites which have a C_7N unit of type (*7.92*) (shown with thickened bonds in the following), namely the mitomycins, e.g. mitomycin B (*7.95*) and ansamycins, e.g. rifamycin S (*7.100*), geldanomycin (*7.99*) and streptovaricin D (*7.101*). So far as examined the C_7N unit does not appear to arise from shikimic acid itself (as the phenazines, Section 7.5.5, with two arguably similar units do) but is deduced to derive from an intermediate a little earlier in the biosynthetic pathway, e.g. dehydroshikimic acid (*7.93*) or dehydroquinic acid (*7.94*) (see Section 5.1).

(7.92)   (7.93)   (7.94)

† The remaining atoms in the mitomycins are derived from citrulline (7.96)/arginine (7.97) and D-glucosamine (7.98): [1-^{13}C, ^{15}N]glucosamine gave mitomycin B (7.95), the mass spectrum of which showed a fragment ion for C-1, C-2, C-3, and N-1a plus attached methyl group, with both stable isotopes present, indicating intact incorporation [48].

(7.95) Mitomycin B

(7.96) X = O
(7.97) X = NH

(7.98)

† The pattern of precursor units in geldanomycin (7.99) follows clearly from experiments with [^{13}C]-labelled precursors. A sequence is indicated of acetate, propionate (not acetate + methyl from methionine) and glycerate units from C-14 through C-1, see (7.99) [49].

† Mixed acetate–propionate pathways (but not including glycerate in the chain) have been deduced for rifamycin S (7.100) and streptovaricin D (7.101). It seems likely that the streptovaricins and rifamycins

(7.99) Geldanomycin

CH_3CO_2H
$HOCH_2CO_2H$
$CH_3CH_2CO_2H$

(7.100) Rifamycin S

(7.101) Streptovaricin D

derive from a common intermediate [50, 51]. The pattern deduced [see (7.102)] for rifamycin S (7.100) has two unusual features: loss of the propionate-derived methyl group from C-28 and insertion of an oxygen between C-12 and C-29 of the precursor. Isolation of rifamycin W with unmodified skeleton, its biosynthesis according to pattern

(*7.102*) and its ready biotransformation into rifamycin B [as (*7.100*) with oxygen-substituted hydroquinone ring B], confirms the rifamycin S pattern and its being a modification of the more orthodox arrangement in (*7.102*).

(7.102)

(7.103)

† The manner of [1-^{13}C]glucose and [1-^{13}C]glycerate incorporation into the C_7N unit of rifamycin S (*7.100*) indicated that biosynthesis of this unit was from a precursor to shikimic acid and that C-9 and C-10 was the location of a dehydroshikimate (*7.93*) double bond. Michael addition to this double bond, as in (*7.103*), allows completion of the naphthoquinone moiety of rifamycin S in an analogous fashion to the formation of the menaquinones (Section 5.2) [52, 53].

7.6.2   Cytochalasins

† The biologically interesting cytochalasins have an origin in phenylalanine (*7.17*) and a C_{16} polyketide, as for example in cytochalasin D (*7.105*), or a C_{18} polyketide, as for example in cytochalasin B (*7.106*). The chain in (*7.106*) is apparently fragmented by the insertion

Acetate

Nonaketide

Octaketide

(7.104)

(7.105) Cytochalasin D

(7.106) Cytochalasin B

● : C_1 unit from methionine

of an oxygen atom into the polyketide chain. This was proved to be so by showing that deoxaphomin (*7.104*) was a precursor for (*7.106*). It is to be noted that, unlike some of the metabolites mentioned above, methionine plus acetate, rather than propionate, serve as precursors for the C_3 units [54].

7.6.3 Nybomycin

† The biosynthesis of nybomycin (*7.107*) has been revealed particularly by use of [1-^{13}C]acetate: C-4, C-6, C-8 and C-10 were found to be labelled and each to an equal extent. The exterior atoms of each

(*7.107*) Nybomycin

pyridone ring therefore are formed from identical acetate-derived C_4 units ([2-^{14}C]acetate could be shown to label C-6′ and C-8′). Methionine is the source of C-2 and C-11′. The origin of the central ring is possibly shikimate or a close relative [55].

7.6.4 Prodiginines

† Particularly clear information on the biogenetic origins of prodigiosin (*7.110*) was obtained by use of [^{13}C]-labelled precursors. This tripyr-role, it turned out, is constituted in the unprecedented way shown (Scheme 7.8). Similar origins have been found for rings A and B of two other metabolites, (*7.111*) and (*7.112*). In ring C there are marked differences between (*7.110*) and the other two metabolites. Appropri-ately the origins are different (Scheme 7.8).

Scheme 7.8

† The aldehyde (7.109) condenses with (7.108) in the ultimate step of prodigiosin (7.110) biosynthesis. It seems probable that (7.109) is a precursor for (7.111) and (7.112) also [56,57].

7.6.5   β-Lactams [60, 61]

Attention must be turned finally to the crucially important penicillins and cephalosporins. They, the nocardicins, e.g. nocardicin A (7.113), and clavulanic acid (7.114) have a β-lactam ring as a common feature. [The deduced origins of (7.113) are shown [58]; (7.114) derives from glycerol (3 units) and probably ketoglutarate [59].]

(7.113) Nocardicin A

L-Serine

L-Homoserine

(7.114) Clavulanic acid

L-Tyrosine

L-Cysteine

L-Valine

(7.115) Penicillin

The penicillins [(7.115); various R groups] and cephalosporins, e.g. cephalosporin C (7.116), are derived from valine (D- and L-isomers equally effective) and cysteine (L-isomer preferred to D). For cephalosporin origins see (7.116). Valine is incorporated into penicillins without nitrogen loss but hydrogen is lost from C-2. DL-[3-^{14}C, ^{15}N, ^{35}S]cystine gave penicillin with the same isotope ratio indicating an intact incorporation. Little hydrogen isotope is lost from C-2 of cysteine. Carbon atom 5 arises from C-3 of cysteine and in the course of biosynthesis of both (7.115) and (7.116) the (3-pro-S)-hydrogen atom of the amino acid is lost. The transformation thus occurs with overall retention of stereochemistry at C-3, and it is interesting to note that if oxidation of the C-3 thio-group to, say, a thiocarbaldehyde occurs in the course of biosynthesis, then the stereochemistry is of the opposite sense to that normally observed in the enzymatic conversion of primary alcohols into aldehydes. The α-aminoadipoyl side chain of (7.116) appears to arise from 2-oxoglutarate plus acetyl coenzyme A [62–65].

The enzymes involved in penicillin and cephalosporin biosynthesis distinguish between the two diastereotopic methyl groups in valine: the

(7.116) Cephalosporin C

(7.117) Penicillin N

● : Me $^{13}CO_2H$
■ : ^{13}Me CO_2H
▲ : $Me_2CHCH(NH_2)$ $^{13}CO_2H$ ⎫
✳ : Me_2CH $^{13}CH(NH_2)CO_2H$ ⎬ Valine
　　　　　　　　　　　　　　　　⎭

(7.118)

(7.119)　　　　　　　　　(7.120)

(*pro-R*)-methyl group (chiral ^{13}C labelling) provides C-2 of (*7.116*) and the β-methyl group of (*7.115*). Deuterium labelling showed that penicillin formation occurred without proton loss from the methyl groups, and two out of the three protons on the (*pro-R*)-methyl group are retained at C-2 in cephalosporin formation (such a result excludes a $\Delta^{2,3}$-cepham intermediate) [66, 67].

Careful work with cell-free systems has shown that penicillin N (*7.117*) with α-aminoadipoyl side-chain is formed, clearly as the first penicillin, from the naturally occurring tripeptide, (*7.118*). [During biosynthesis precursor L-valine suffers inversion of configuration on formation of (*7.118*); inversion of configuration in the α-aminoadipoyl residue in (*7.118*) occurs on conversion into (*7.117*).] Penicillin N (*7.117*) in turn serves as a precursor for cephalosporin C (*7.116*) [68, 69].

The above results closely define the fates of individual atoms and the stereochemistry of reactions involved in penicillin/cephalosporin biosynthesis as well as indicating the pathway followed. What remains unknown are the mechanisms of the two ring-closure reactions from (*7.118*). There are, however, several attractive possibilities, for β-lactam formation at least. One suggestion is that cyclization occurs by a variation of the ene reaction; see (*7.119*). This is an alternative to the simpler idea of nucleophilic attack of amide nitrogen on the sp^2 carbon of a thioaldehyde or its sp^3 receptor equivalent. A quite different possibility is that cyclization is associated with oxidation of the amide nitrogen; nucleophilic displacement at this centre by an anion generated at the β-carbon of the cysteine fragment follows; see

(*7.120*) [70, 71]. In so far as any of these mechanisms depend particularly on the presence of sulphur they are likely to be incorrect, since the only assistance available for β-lactam formation in clavulanic acid (*7.114*) or nocardicin A (*7.113*) is from oxygen. Shutting the penicillin thiazole ring is likely to involve the generation and coupling of radicals.

References

Further reading: *Biosynthesis (Specialist Periodical Reports)* [ed. T. A. Geissman (vols. 1–3), ed. J. D. Bu'Lock (vols. 4 and 5)], The Chemical Society, London; Herbert, R. B. in *The Alkaloids (Specialist Periodical Reports)* [ed. J. E. Saxton (vols. 1–5), ed. M. F. Grundon (vols. 6–10)], The Chemical Society, London; [1].

[1] Herbert, R. B. (1980), in *Rodd's Chemistry of Carbon Compounds*, 2nd Edn, (ed. S. Coffey), Elsevier, Amsterdam, vol. IV L, pp. 291–455.
[2] Guengerich, F. P., Snyder, J. J. and Broquist, H. P. (1973), *Biochemistry*, **12**, 4264–9.
[3] Bach, M. L. and Gilvarg, C. (1966), *J. Biol. Chem.*, **241**, 4563–4.
[4] Kanie, M., Fujimoto, S. and Foster, J. W. (1966), *J. Bact.*, **91**, 570–7.
[5] Terashima, T., Idaka, E., Kishi, Y. and Goto, T. (1973), *J. Chem. Soc. Chem. Comm.*, 75–6.
[6] Dobson, T. A., Desaty, D., Brewer, D. and Vining, L. C. (1967), *Can. J. Biochem.*, **45**, 809–23.
[7] Helbling, A. M. and Viscontini, M. (1976), *Helv. Chim. Acta*, **59**, 2284–9.
[8] Wright, J. L. C., Vining, L. C., McInnes, A. G., Smith, D. G. and Walter, J. A. (1977), *Can. J. Biochem.*, **55**, 678–85.
[9] Leete, E., Kowanko, N., Newmark, R. A., Vining, L. C., McInnes, A. G. and Wright, J. L. C. (1975), *Tetrahedron Lett.*, 4103–6.
[10] Iwai, Y., Kumano, K. and Omura, S. (1978), *Chem. Pharm. Bull. (Japan)*, **26**, 736–9.
[11] Birch, A. J. and Simpson, T. J. (1979), *J. Chem. Soc. Perkin I*, 816–22.
[12] Vining, L. C. and Wright, J. L. C. (1977), in *Biosynthesis (Specialist Periodical Reports)* (ed. J. D. Bu'Lock), The Chemical Society, London, vol. 5, pp. 240–305.
[13] Allen, C. M., jun. (1973), *J. Amer. Chem. Soc.*, **95**, 2386–7.
[14] Marchelli, R., Dossena, A. and Casnati, G. (1975), *J. Chem. Soc. Chem. Comm.*, 779–80.
[15] Baldas, J., Birch, A. J. and Russell, R. A. (1974), *J. Chem. Soc. Perkin I*, 50–2.
[16] MacDonald, J. C. and Slater, G. P. (1975), *Can. J. Biochem.*, **53**, 475–8.
[17] Kirby, G. W. and Narayanaswami, S. (1976), *J. Chem. Soc. Perkin I*, 1564–7.
[18] MacDonald, J. C. (1965), *Biochem. J.*, **96**, 533–8.
[19] Akers, H. A., Llinás, M. and Nielands, J. B. (1972), *Biochemistry*, **11**, 2283–91.
[20] Hanke, T. and Diekmann, H. (1974), *Arch. Microbiol.*, **95**, 227–36.

[21] Barrow, K. D., Colley, P. W. and Tribe, D. E. (1979), *J. Chem. Soc. Chem. Comm.*, 225–6.
[22] Kirby, G. W., Patrick, G. L. and Robins, D. J. (1978), *J. Chem. Soc. Perkin I*, 1336–8.
[23] Kirby, G. W. and Varley, M. J. (1974), *J. Chem. Soc. Chem. Comm.*, 833–4.
[24] Aboutabl, El S. A., El Azzouny, A., Winter, K. and Luckner, M. (1976), *Phytochemistry*, **15**, 1925–8.
[25] Chang, C., Floss, H. G., Hurley, L. H. and Zmijewski, M. (1976), *J. Org. Chem.*, **41**, 2932–4.
[26] Hurley, L. H., Gairola, C. and Das, N. V. (1976), *Biochemistry*, **15**, 3760–9.
[27] Floss, H. G. (1976), *Tetrahedron*, **32**, 873–912.
[28] Lee, S.-L., Floss, H. G. and Heinstein, P. (1976), *Arch. Biochem. Biophys.*, **177**, 84–94.
[29] Plieninger, H., Meyer, E., Maier, W. and Gröger, D. (1978), *Annalen*, 813–7.
[30] Floss, H. G., Tcheng-Lin, M., Chang, C., Naidoo, B., Blair, G. E., Abou-Chaar, C. I. and Cassady, J. M. (1974), *J. Amer. Chem. Soc.*, **96**, 1898–909.
[31] Abe, M. (1970), paper presented at the first International Symposium on Genetics of Industrial Micro-organisms, Prague. (see ref. [27]).
[32] Gröger, D., Mothes, K., Floss, H. G. and Weygand, F. (1963), *Z. Naturforsch.*, **18b**, 1123–4.
[33] Gröger, D., Johne, S. and Härtling, S. (1974), *Biochem. Physiol. Pflanzen.*, **166**, 33–43.
[34] Floss, H. G., Tcheng-Lin, M., Kobel, H. and Stadler, P. (1974), *Experientia*, **30**, 1369–70.
[35] McGrath, R. M., Stein, P. S., Ferreira, N. P. and Neethling, D. C. (1976), *Bio-org. Chem.*, **5**, 11–23.
[36] Mascaro, L., jun., Hörhammer, R., Eisenstein, S., Sellers, L. K., Mascaro, K. and Floss, H. G. (1977), *J. Amer. Chem. Soc.*, **99**, 273–4.
[37] Gould, S. J. and Darling, D. S. (1978), *Tetrahedron Lett.* 3207–10.
[38] Martin, L. L., Chang, C.-J., Floss, H. G., Mabe, J. A., Hagaman, E. W. and Wenkert, E. (1972), *J. Amer. Chem. Soc.*, **94**, 8942–4.
[39] Salcher, O., Lingens, F. and Fischer, P. (1978), *Tetrahedron Lett.*, 1978, 3097–100.
[40] Ritter, C. and Luckner, M. (1971), *Eur. J. Biochem.*, **18**, 391–400.
[41] Butenandt, A. and Beckmann, R. (1955), *Z. Physiol. Chem.*, **301**, 115–7.
[42] Herbert, R. B. (1974), *Tetrahedron Lett.*, 4525–8.
[43] Etherington, T., Herbert, R. B., Holliman, F. G. and Sheridan, J. B. (1979), *J. Chem. Soc. Perkin I*, 2416–9.
[44] Byng, G. S. and Turner, J. M. (1977), *Biochem. J.*, **164**, 133–45.
[45] Herbert, R. B., Holliman, F. G. and Ibberson, P. N. (1972), *J. Chem. Soc. Chem. Comm.*, 355–6.
[46] Flood, M. E., Herbert, R. B. and Holliman, F. G. (1972), *J. Chem. Soc. Perkin I*, 622–6.
[47] Simonsen, J. N., Paramasigamani, K., Vining, L. C., McInnes, A. G., Walter, J. A. and Wright, J. L. C. (1978), *Can. J. Microbiol.*, **24**, 136–42.

[48] Hornemann, U., Kehrer, J. P. and Eggert, J. H. (1974), *J. Chem. Soc. Chem. Comm.*, 1045–6.

[49] Haber, A., Johnson, R. D. and Rinehart, K. L., jun. (1977), *J. Amer. Chem. Soc.*, **99**, 3541–4.

[50] Milavetz, B., Kakinuma, K., Rinehart, K. L., jun., Rolls, J. P. and Haak, W. J. (1973), *J. Amer. Chem. Soc.*, **95**, 5793–5.

[51] Ghisalba, O., Traxler, P. and Nüesch, J. (1978), *J. Antibiotics*, **31**, 1124–31.

[52] White, R. J. and Martinelli, E. (1974), *FEBS Lett.*, **49**, 233–6.

[53] Ghisalba, O. and Nüesch, J. (1978), *J. Antibiotics*, **31**, 215–25.

[54] Vederas, J. C. and Tamm, C. (1976), *Helv. Chim. Acta*, **59**, 558–66.

[55] Nadzan, A. M. and Rinehart, K. L., jun. (1976), *J. Amer. Chem. Soc.*, **98**, 5012–4.

[56] Wasserman, H. H., Shaw, C. K., Sykes, R. J. and Cushley, R. J. (1974), *Tetrahedron Lett.*, 2787–90.

[57] Gerber, N. N., McInnes, A. G., Smith, D. G., Walter, J. A., Wright, J. L. C. and Vining, L. C. (1978), *Can. J. Chem.*, **56**, 1155–63.

[58] Hosada, J., Tani, N., Konomi, T., Ohsawa, S., Aoki, H. and Imanaka, H. (1977), *Agric. and Biol. Chem. (Japan)*, **41**, 2007–12.

[59] Elson, S. W. and Oliver, R. S. (1978), *J. Antibiotics*, **31**, 586–92.

[60] Flynn, E. H. (ed.) (1972), *Cephalosporins and Penicillins, Chemistry and Biology*, Academic Press, New York.

[61] Aberhart, D. J. (1977), *Tetrahedron*, **33**, 1545–59.

[62] Booth, H., Bycroft, B. W., Wels, C. M., Corbett, K. and Maloney, A. P. (1976), *J. Chem. Soc. Chem. Comm.*, 110–1.

[63] Huddleston, J. A., Abraham, E. P., Young, D. W., Morecombe, D. J. and Sen, P. K. (1978), *Biochem. J.*, **169**, 705–7.

[64] Neuss, N., Nash, C. H., Lemke, P. A. and Grutzner, J. B. (1971), *J. Amer. Chem. Soc.*, **93**, 2337–9.

[65] Neuss, N., Nash, C. H., Lemke, P. A. and Grutzner, J. B. (1971), *Proc. Roy. Soc.*, **B179**, 335–44.

[66] Kluender, H., Huang, F.-C., Fritzberg, A., Schnoes, H., Sih, C. J., Fawcett, P. and Abraham, E. P. (1974), *J. Amer. Chem. Soc.*, **96**, 4054–5.

[67] Aberhart, D. J., Chu, J. Y.-R., Neuss, N., Nash, C. H., Occolowitz, J., Huckstep, L. L. and De La Higura, N. (1974), *J. Chem. Soc. Chem. Comm.*, 564–5.

[68] Fawcett, P. A., Usher, J. J., Huddleston, J. A., Bleaney, R. C., Nisbet, J. J. and Abraham, E. P. (1976), *Biochem. J.*, **157**, 651–60.

[69] Khosata, M. and Demain, A. L. (1976), *Biochem. Biophys. Res. Comm.*, **70**, 465–73.

[70] Scott, A. I., Yoo, S. E., Chung, S.-K. and Lacadie, J. A. (1976), *Tetrahedron Lett.* 1137–40.

[71] Cheney, J., Moores, C. J., Raleigh, J. A., Scott, A. I. and Young, D. W. (1974), *J. Chem. Soc. Chem. Comm.*, 47–8.

Index